FIT NOT FAT AFTER 50

A 50-STEP GUIDE TO HEALTH, FITNESS AND WEIGHT LOSS, THAT PROVES OVER-50 DOESN'T HAVE TO MEAN OVER THE HILL

By
Aylia Fox

FIT NOT FAT AFTER 50

Copyright © Aylia Fox, 2021

All rights reserved.

No part of this book may be reproduced by any means, nor transmitted, nor translated into a machine language, without the written permission of the publishers.

Aylia Fox has asserted her right to be identified as the author of this work in accordance with sections 77 and 78 of the Copyright, Designs and Patents Act 1988.

Condition of Sale

This book is sold subject to the condition that it shall not, by way of trade or otherwise, be lent, re-sold, hired out or otherwise circulated in any form of binding or cover other than that in which it is published and without a similar condition including this condition being imposed on the subsequent purchaser.

ISBN: 978-1-80049-522-7

"Age is an issue of mind over matter.

If you don't mind, it doesn't matter"

Mark Twain

CONTENTS

Introduction..7

Part One
DIET, FOOD & WEIGHT LOSS........................17

Part Two
EXERCISE..45

Part Three
THE MIND AND MENTAL HEALTH................101

Part Four
LIFESTYLE...119

Afterword...127

INTRODUCTION

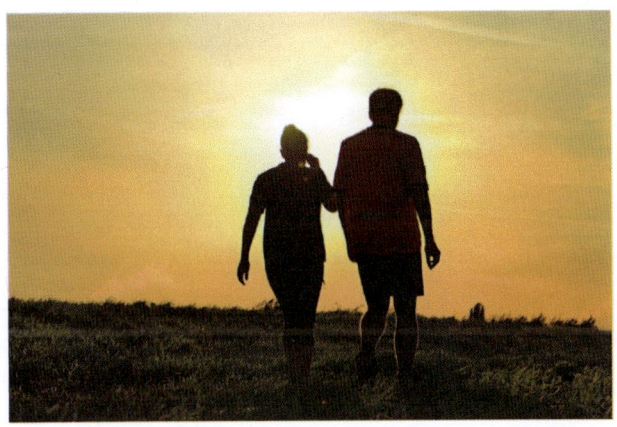

This is NOT a book for old people. This is NOT a book about getting old. If it was, I would start by listing all the unpleasant things that can happen to your body once you've reached your half century.

But that would be depressing, and I do it later anyway. No, this is a book for people who just happen to be over the age of 50 who want a health and fitness guide tailored to them – just as you can tailor a health and fitness guide to other categories of people such as pregnant women, those with an injury or children.

This is also a book for people who believe age is just a number and if that number happens to be 50+, that shouldn't *necessarily* mean that everything changes in terms of health and fitness.

I am one of those believers. I'm nearly 56 and I've never been fitter or healthier. I have a metabolic age of 29, my cardiovascular fitness is much better than women half my age who exercise, and I'm stronger than any of the men I've ever worked with as a personal trainer. I've never taken a day off work through illness, my weight is in the 'excellent' range for my height and my build is described as 'slim athletic.' None of this is down to luck or good genes, it's down to hard work, commitment, consistency, a bit of sacrifice and an ongoing desire to achieve goals.

I'm not a narcissist or show off. I simply want you to know that it's possible to be super-fit and healthy when you're NOT young.

A warning though: if you're new to health, fitness and weight loss, you should consult your GP before embarking on a new regime. And, once given the thumbs-up, don't try to do too much too soon and don't expect too much right away. This has got nothing to do with age, it's just that the body needs time to adjust to a new regime and then adapt in order to facilitate change.

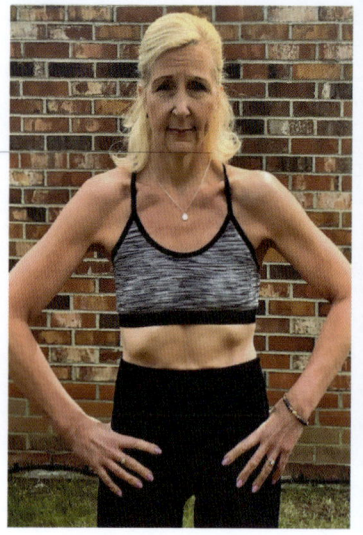

Aylia Fox

This is not an overnight process and you need to establish a pattern of new behaviours which are sustainable — a process which, by definition, takes time.

That's not an excuse to introduce one tiny change at a time though. Be realistic: you're over 50, time's not on your side and if you want to see improvements as quickly as is practical, I suggest you throw yourself into your new plan wholeheartedly. If this means making several simultaneous changes, then that's what you should do.

Fortunately, you're likely to have more years on the planet than your parents or grandparents. According to the World Health Organisation, "The pace of population ageing around the world is increasing dramatically. A longer life brings with it great opportunities...yet the extent of these opportunities depends heavily on one factor: health."

The Office for National Statistics reports that in 1950, 5.3 million people in the UK were aged 65 or over. Today, that figure is in excess of 12 million and for 2050, the over-65 population prediction is 17.1 million.

And, in case you're wondering, if you're a woman you can currently expect to live to around the age of 86; and if you're a man, it's 83.5.

So unless you get run down by a bus, you've got a shot at long life - and if you want to enjoy the retirement of your dreams, spend quality years with your grandkids and do it all with a smile on your face because you're fit and healthy, read on.

Coming up is no-nonsense, practical advice in terms of things you should and shouldn't do on your health and fitness journey. It's a guide with a mission but it's not sugar coated. Expect unpalatable facts about the process — and if you take up the challenges I set you, plan for a few setbacks along the way.

In short, if you're new to health and fitness and want to reach your potential, you'll have to push yourself physically AND manage your mind to give you psychological strength.

Any book can tell you to eat less and move more — it sounds simple and in some respects it is, but if you've ever been on a diet before, you'll know there's a lot more to weight loss (and weight gain) than that. In fact, the entire process is played out in the mind (see Part 3).

It's not easy controlling how and what you eat; it's hard finding the willpower to subdue food cravings. It's tough walking into a gym for the first time and it's even tougher tolerating the discomfort of exercise on a regular basis.

So, right from the outset, I recommend you learn how to harness the power of your mind in order to influence your reality.

Think positively, believe in yourself, manifest outcomes and refer to Mark Twain's 'mind over matter' quote at the beginning of the book — which essentially means that if you give your mind permission to be your controlling authority, you can achieve anything.

Mind you, you'll still have to work harder than someone in their 20's, 30's or even 40's…

And the reason for this? Well, unfortunately, there are certain physiological changes that take place at around the age of 50 that you simply cannot avoid. None of them are good and all of them make it more difficult to achieve health and fitness goals.

Harder, but possible. Cling to that phrase without the 'harder' bit and you'll be fine. I'm going to show you how in **50 simple steps.**

Many of those 50 steps are guiding principles that can be used and modified whatever your age. So even if you're in your 20s, carry on reading, you too can reap the rewards.

The book is divided into three main sections which relate to the three core components of overall health and fitness.

- **Part 1: Diet, food, and weight loss**
- **Part 2: Exercise**
- **Part 3: The mind and mental health**

One area is no more important than the other because they work symbiotically. What this means is that benefits from one area trigger benefits from another in a chain reaction I have labelled the **Tri-Hybrid-Health**© model.

Most people tend to focus on one area — the most common being weight loss. However, what they fail to realise is that this approach ignores the many other factors that go hand in hand with successful and sustainable weight loss — i.e. exercise and mind/mental health.

Overall health is like a jigsaw — there's many pieces that need to fit together for a successful outcome. **Tri-Hybrid-Health**© recognises this and focusses on the three key areas that make up the bigger picture.

If you're looking for overall health and fitness you should give each of the sections equal attention. One is no more important than the other because they work symbiotically.

But why bother with all this effort and exertion I hear you ask? Well, the benefits of being fit, healthy and not overweight are numerous and well documented, but I'll summarise them for you:

- You will live longer
- You will be less prone to disease and better able to fight it
- You will have improved mental health
- You will feel younger
- You will look better

Trust me, I know what I'm talking about — and not just from personal experience. I've worked as a certified personal trainer for many years and had hundreds of clients of varying ages and abilities — including people in the public eye. Many of them have been over the age of 50.

But one thing all clients have in common is this: if they train hard and achieve their goals, then health and fitness transforms their life. They become an improved version of their former selves, both physically and mentally.

I once worked with an actress who was due to appear on the TV show I'm A Celebrity Get Me Out of Here. She wanted a bikini-ready body in order to impress, and she worked hard to achieve one. Unfortunately, she had to pull out of the show at the last minute but went on to front a number of fitness DVDs which sold well. It was clear to me she'd caught what I like to call the 'exercise bug' and I now enjoy watching her on-screen promoting health and fitness, as she does regularly.

I'm also the former Medical Correspondent of a national newspaper and can draw on years of experience of writing and researching stories about health, fitness, medicine and science.

I once interviewed the Secretary of State for Health at the time, William Waldegrave, who told me:

"Aylia, are you aware that the greatest wealth is health?"

I was young, nonchalant and rather cynical back then, and I recall raising my eyebrows. I suspected he was talking in soundbites for the sake of the story. Now I'm in my mid 50's I get it. He was right.

I've learned many things along the way but the best bit of advice I can give your right now is the following: health and fitness is not a magic wand; it won't solve all your problems, but it's the nearest damned thing you've got to one and you don't have to be Harry Houdini to cast an amazing spell over yourself.

So, if you don't want to be fat and unfit after 50 — and become a victim of the consequential problems — you CAN do something about it. And it's never too late to start. The benefits are up for grabs whether you're 25, 55 or 95. And the sooner you start, the sooner you'll thank yourself for doing so.

ANATOMICAL PRELUDE: THE AGEING PROCESS

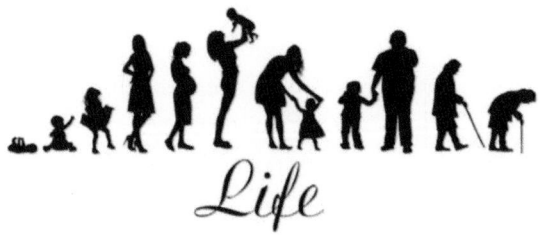

As we age, so does the internal workings of the body. Everything slows down; It's how evolution works. No one can live forever and once our reproductive duties are complete and we've raised our young, our biological reason for existing is over. Brutal but true.
Chronologically, this slowing process kicks-in at around the age of 50.

We can't stop it, but we can fight it and mitigate the effect of the changes by boosting our health and fitness.

What this means is controlling our weight by controlling our diet and keeping metabolically fit through exercise. Add mind/mental health into the mix, and you're well onto your way to optimum health. The focus of the book is how to achieve this, but first some information about exactly what those age-related changes are and what they mean on an everyday basis. In general, ageing is the gradual but steady erosion of the body's organ systems and of its in-built capacity to repair itself. Specifically it is:

CHANGES IN BODY COMPOSITION

The structural elements of tissue mutate the longer we live. This leads to several things, including a higher proportion of body fat and a lower level of water content. The increased body fat combined with a slowing of the metabolic rate (the speed at which calories are burned) often leads to weight gain — particularly around the abdomen. When the body lacks enough water, cells become 'sticky' 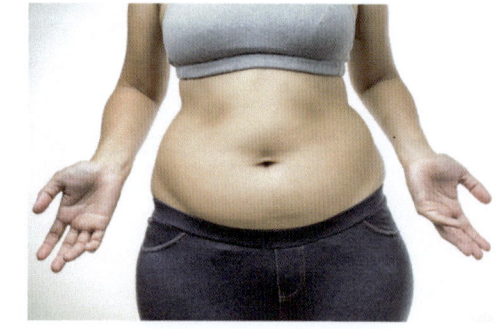 which slows the movement of blood and oxygen and can adversely affect our breathing and our ability to remove waste products.

HORMONES

Hormonal change in middle age influences many things including the loss of lean muscle mass and a decrease in bone density. Losing muscle makes us weaker and causes fatigue while bones soften and lose their pliability and become brittle — hence older people tend to have more falls and their bones break more easily than a young person's.

Hormones are also responsible for the onset of menopause in women, during which the ovaries stop producing eggs and the level of the hormones oestrogen and progesterone decrease. The side effects of this are numerous and can affect women in different ways. However, many experience mood swings, irritability, hot flushes, night sweats, brain fog, insomnia, anxiety, decreased libido, fatigue and weight gain. Some men develop similar symptoms at around the same age which is sometimes described as the male menopause. Although it's a fact that the male sex hormone testosterone decreases as a man ages, the medical jury's out on whether it's an official condition.

THE HEART

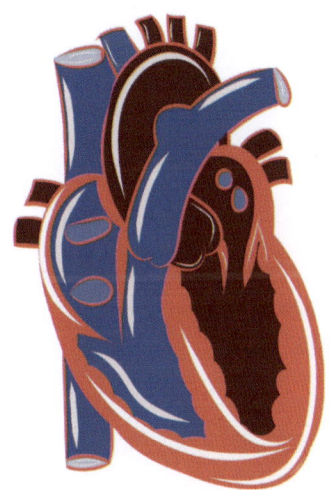

We can compare the heart to a car engine — as the engine gets older and has more use, it becomes worn and tired and eventually conks out. With a car it can be replaced with a new one, but unless you qualify for a heart transplant because you have a life threatening condition, there's not a lot you can do about it. The heart is responsible for pumping the blood around the body and this effects the capacity of our lungs to generate oxygen for physical use. Also, the tubes in the lungs narrow and break down whereby oxygen flow is slower. If the body doesn't get enough oxygen or the heart stops working properly, you're in trouble.

THE JOINTS

A joint is the connection between two bones which link up to make the skeletal system. With age and use, the cushioning and lubricating matter between them e.g., cartilage — wears out.

This causes inflammation and pain and often leads to movement reduction. Examples of two common and serious joint conditions are osteoarthritis and rheumatoid arthritis. Neither can be cured, only treated.

Other ageing changes include:

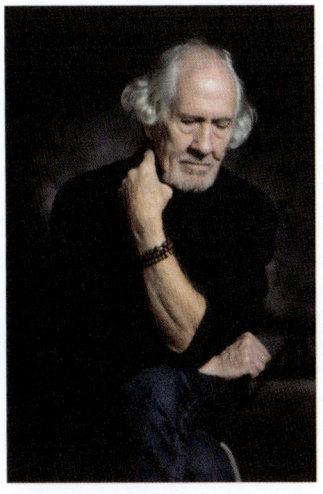

FAILING EYESIGHT

The eye contains muscle which, like any other muscle in the body, deteriorates with age and use.

Age-related macular degeneration is a common condition mainly affecting people in their 50's or 60's. Characterised by a loss of vision in the middle part of the eye, it makes reading and recognising faces difficult. Aside from age, it's been linked to high blood pressure, smoking and being overweight.

Cataracts is a serious eye condition that causes the lens of your eye to go cloudy. It can lead to blindness and is often age related or connected to diabetes.

DECREASED MEMORY RECALL

As we age, brain cells die. Those responsible for short term memory tend to die first.

This may mean you forget what somebody just said to you or you go into a room and forget why.

CHANGES IN SKIN

Collagen - the main building block of skin and connective tissue — decreases leading to sagging skin and wrinkles. This is most noticeable on the face.

CHANGES IN HAIR

Hair goes grey due to the loss of pigment. It also thins and fall out due to hormonal changes and vitamin and mineral deficiencies (the body absorbs them less effectively the older you get).

SHRINKING STATURE

As we age, the discs between our vertebrae dry and thin, which leads to spinal compression. Poor posture is an additional cause.

DECREASED BLADDER CONTROL

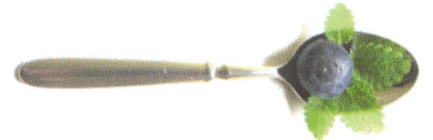

With age, the muscles in our pelvis weaken, which can lead to urinary incontinence.

DIGESTIVE PROBLEMS

The oesophagus and bowel slow down as you get older which affects the intestines and digestion. This has numerous knock-on effects such as constipation.

All these conditions and ailments can happen to normal, healthy people who are not overweight. But, if you're unhealthy, unfit and overweight, they're more likely to happen to you AND one of the following life-threatening conditions too:

- Heart disease (which can lead to heart attack/failure)
- Type 2 Diabetes
- Stroke
- Some cancers (colon, breast, oesophagus)
- High Blood pressure
- High cholesterol
- Breathing problems such as sleep apnoea and asthma
- Early onset dementia
- Gall Bladder Disease (including gallstones)
- Numerous circulatory diseases such as Pulmonary
- Embolism (a blood clot on the lung)
- Lymphedema (severe localised fluid retention)

Other unwelcome conditions you may develop include ulcers (of the stomach and skin), hernia, acid reflux, urinary incontinence, insomnia, general aches and pains (particularly in the back) headaches and migraines, panic attacks and some mental health conditions such as depression.

That's a lot of scary things you really want to avoid. So, if you're fat, unfit, over 50 and want to reduce your chances of getting them, the first thing you need to do is lose weight.

PART ONE

DIET, FOOD AND WEIGHT LOSS

This section — and the beginning of the 50-point guide – will focus on Diet, nutrition, weight loss and associated topics which will be of use on your health and fitness journey.

So, how do you know if you need to lose weight? Well, there's several tests you can do yourself which will give you a very good idea.

1
CALCULATE YOUR BODY MASS INDEX

BMI is a scale of numbers used by doctors to determine a patient's weight status. The formula used to determine your BMI is:

Your weight in kgs divided by your height in metres squared.

For example, if you're 75 kg and you're 1.75 metres tall, you multiply 1.75 by itself and divide the answer (3.06) into 75. The total in this case is 24.5

A healthy BMI is within the range of 18.5-24.9 (men and women)
You don't have to do the maths yourself, there are many online resources that do it for you and most digital scales display it when you weigh yourself.

So now you have a number, all you need to do is refer to the following table to find out what your status is:

BMI of under 16: severely underweight
BMI of less than 18.5: underweight
BMI of 18.5-24.9: healthy weight
BMI of 25 – 29.9: overweight
BMI of 30 - 34.9: obese class 1
BMI of 35 – 39.9: obese class 2
BMI of 40+: morbidly obese

Apart from your weight and BMI, the other important figure relating to body composition that you need to know is your body fat %.

2
CHECK YOUR BODY FAT PERCENTAGE

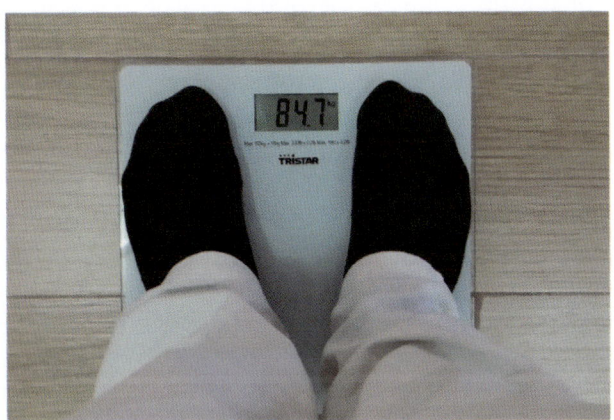

There's really only one way to determine this from the comfort of your own home and that is to invest in a set of body analyser digital scales. Prices start at around £12.

Make sure you read the information about the product before you buy, because some digital scales only read your weight.

The term to look for on the packaging is '*body analyser*'. In addition to your weight and BMI, they will also record your body fat % and other useful statistics such as your hydration level, your muscle mass, your bone mass, and your Basal Metabolic Rate – the daily number of calories your body requires to sustain itself.

The scales work by sending a tiny electrical impulse through your body (you don't feel a thing) which measures your body's resistance to it.

If you are overweight, it is likely that your body fat % will be out of the healthy range. Even if you are a healthy weight, your body fat % can be high. The same goes for underweight people - a phenomenon known as 'skinny-fat'.

Having an unhealthy body fat level is a problem because it can lead to one or more of the chronic diseases that are also associated with being overweight, e.g. heart disease and Type 2 Diabetes.

Body fat is stored in two different ways – fat that you can see, e.g. on your abdomen, thighs, or face. This is known as subcutaneous. Fat that you cannot see internally that is known as visceral. This is more of a threat because it surrounds vital organs such as your heart, liver and pancreas and can prevent them from working properly.

Once you have a figure for your body fat %, use the following table to determine whether you need to do anything about it.

The lower the percentage, the better (within reason, of course; the body needs some fat to function properly and there are serious risks associated with an extremely low level):

Aged 50-59	**Healthy**	**Above Average**	**High**
Female	35% or less	35.1-40%	Over 40%
Male	22% or less	22.1-28%	Over 28%

Aged 60-80	**Healthy**	**Above Average**	**High**
Female	36% or less	36.1-42%	Over 42%
Male	25% or less	25.1-30%	Over 30%

3

MEASURE YOUR WAIST AND HIPS

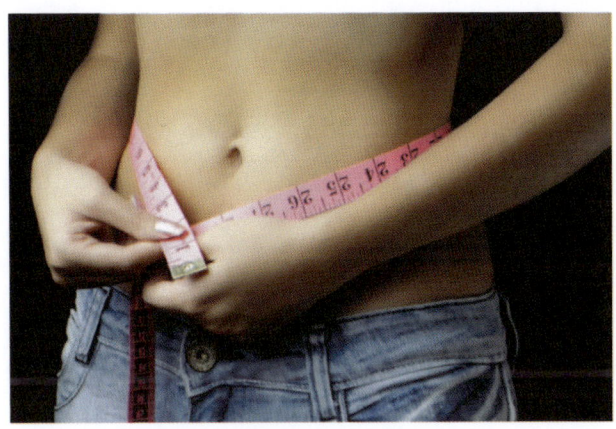

Carrying a greater proportion of your weight/fat around your abdomen rather than your hips means a greater chance of health problems. This is because of its proximity to vital organs such as the heart and kidney. Fat isn't static. It can 'seep' into nearby organs causing damage. Also, the extra weight in that area can put undue pressure on the heart and lead to problems such as high blood pressure, heart attack and stroke.

If you carry most of your weight round your middle, you can be described as apple shaped (this mainly applies to women).

Carrying your weight around your hips and thighs is described as pear shaped.

Doctors often look to the size of your waist as an indicator of potential for health issues. You want your waist to measure less than your hips and the ratio between the two is even more important.

Women should aim for a waist circumference of less than 80 cm and men less than 94. If your waist measurement is more than 88 cm for a woman and 102 cm for a man, then your risk of health problems significantly increases. A recent study showed that women with an unhealthy waist size were 30 per cent more likely to get breast cancer for example.

To calculate your ratio, simply divide your waist circumference by your hip's circumference.

A ratio of more than 0.85 for women and 1.0 for men means you're carrying too much weight around your middle.

For example: someone who has a waist measurement of 76 and a hip measurement of 97 has a ratio of 0.78.

If you've got a big belly, you're not alone. The average waist size for a woman in Britain is 84.3 cm and for a man, it's 96.3 cm. The average dress size for a woman is size 16. Just because it's average, doesn't make it right!

If you discover you need to lose weight and/or body fat, the next thing to do is:

4
SET TARGETS

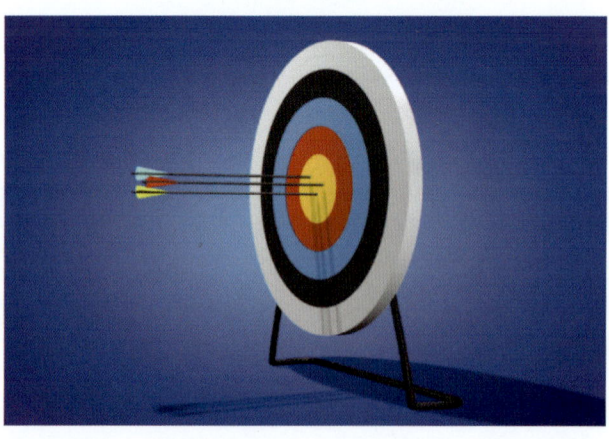

You are more likely to make lasting changes if you set yourself goals. Ideally have short, medium and long term ones so that each feels achievable.

Write down the goals and tell people what you're doing. This should be motivating because it makes you accountable. In the case of losing weight, it's not unwise to have an approximate target weight, but I strongly recommend you don't fixate on the numbers on the scales.

Think outside the box – maybe you'd really prefer to go down a dress size or you might decide it's best for you to monitor your body fat percentage.

You could, perhaps, set nutrition goals – such as only having healthy snacks between meals or ensuring you have breakfast every morning.

Whatever you want to achieve, that should be your goal.

Or here's a radical thought – why not just concentrate on what your body can do, rather than what it weighs or what it looks like? Assuming you start some serious exercise, you'll soon be amazed at what it's capable of. The pay offs will almost certainly include the thing you once assumed was your goal – for example weight loss.

Whatever you decide your targets are, you should record starting points against which you can compare your progress as you advance – begin with the ones listed above, weight, BMI, body fat %.

5

ASSESS YOUR CURRENT DIET

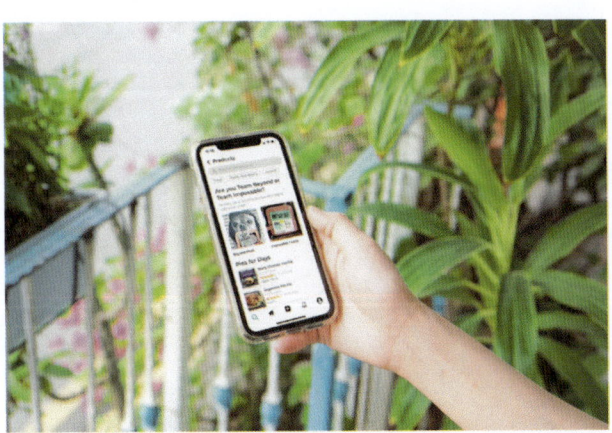

One of the most effective ways to do this is to keep a food diary for an average week. Log down everything you eat and drink and take a long, hard look at it. If it's full of junk food, fat, sugar and salt, then it's unhealthy. If fruit, veg, salad, whole-grains and fibre are lacking, it's even unhealthier and if you drink more than the recommended units of alcohol per week, snack on calorific food between meals and enjoy massive portions then it's a nutrition disaster.

Next, it's worthwhile calculating your current calorie consumption to determine where you stand on the suitability of your intake. Either do this manually by reading labels and doing calculations, or better still, there are numerous online resources and tracker apps which do it for you.

Some of the popular ones include: the NHS website, MyFitnessPal, FitBit, Lose It! and FatSecret. An ideal intake of calories depends on your age, your activity level, and your metabolism, but generally **the recommendation for a man is between 2,000-2,500 a day and for a woman it's 1,500-2,000.**

6

CHANGE YOUR DIET DON'T GO ON A DIET

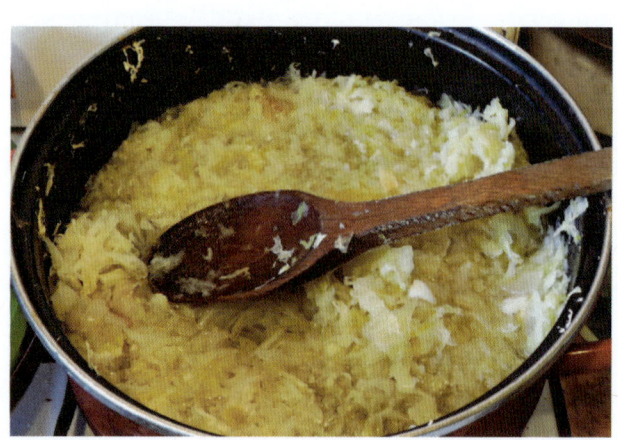

It's generally accepted by those in-the-know, that diets don't work – not long term anyway. The vast majority are unsustainable and the vital thing about effective weight loss (particularly after the age of 50) is that it needs to be long term to have any fundamental effects. How would you choose a diet anyway?

There is an avalanche of misinformation out there, along with thousands of diets, all making the same basic assertion - that theirs is the best and, in most cases, the quickest to see results. Most make unfounded claims in terms of how much weight you can expect to lose in a certain amount of time, and many are compiled by people with no medical, health or fitness credentials. Then you've got your fad diets. Popular ones include: the cabbage soup diet, the grapefruit diet, the South Beach Diet, The Caveman Diet, the Zone Diet, The Cookie Diet, The Blood Group Diet and The Hollywood 48-hour Miracle Diet. Also, there's the meal replacement diets; the cutting-out of a food group diets and the so-called fasting diets.

But the one thing almost all diets have in common, is that they involve deprivation of one sort of another. With deprivation comes misery and with misery comes obsession. You end up craving all the things you're banned from eating, and when that feeling gets overwhelming (as it inevitably will for most people) you give up. A few days/weeks/months later you start another diet, and the same thing happens until you give up altogether and find you weigh more than you did at the beginning of the process. It's known as yo-yo dieting and some people spend their life doing it, but never lose weight long term.

7
BECOME CALORIE CONSCIOUS

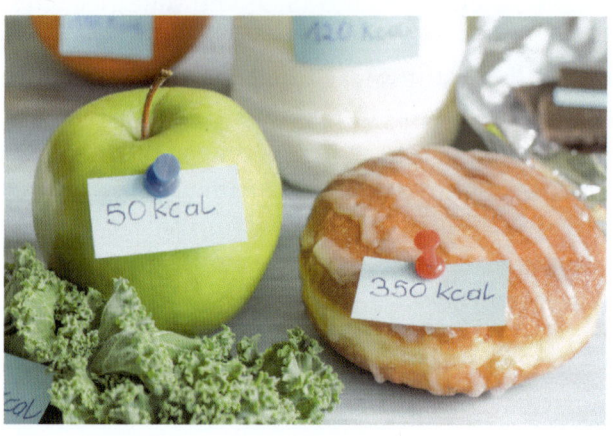

Calorie counting is considered rather old fashioned nowadays. But there is a simple physiological fact that underpins all weight loss, and that is: **if you eat fewer calories than you burn – on a consistent basis – you will lose weight. This is known as calorie deficit.** The reverse is true and, if you eat the same amount as you burn, you're likely to maintain weight.

Therefore, I don't believe calories should be ignored. I think they should be acknowledged as relevant components in a weight loss plan, but only to the extent where you're sentient and sensible around them.

So how many calories *should* you have?

There is not a one-size-fits-all method for calorie counting because much depends on your activity level and your weight in the first place but there are minimum levels. **An average woman shouldn't drop below around 1,200 a day and for a man it's around 1,700.**

As previously mentioned, if you choose to count calories it's easy to do so with a wide variety of online and app tracker resources in which you can also monitor your activity levels to get an overall picture of your calorie deficit.

The other useful thing about being calorie conscious is that it gives you the freedom to decide how to divide your food and drink throughout the day. Also, no food or food groups are banned, and none are singled out (imagine eating cabbage soup for a week!) And, with a bit of imagination and planning, you can include your favourite foods, have the odd gin and tonic and dine out from time to time.

That's not to say you shouldn't maintain good nutrition – you should – and I urge you take a look at the NHS's Eat well Plate which demonstrates, by dividing up a plate, the proportions of foods you should be eating for good health.

If, however, one day you get up and decide you want a chocolate bar for breakfast, lunch, and dinner, if it's within the calorie allowance you've given yourself, then why not?! **(this is not recommended!)**

And if you overdo it calorie-wise one day, you can choose to cut back a bit the following day.

Being calorie conscious still works for a lot of people and if it works for you, there's no reason not to do it.

Below is an example of what a woman could eat and drink on an average day incorporating three meals and two snacks for around **1,300 calories:**

Breakfast: Two eggs — either boiled, scrambled, or poached, 1 turkey medallion, 3 tablespoons of low sugar baked beans and a piece of fruit e.g. an orange
(approx. 300 calories)

Lunch: Bowl of healthy or low-cal soup, 1 slice of Danish-style bread with low fat spread and a low fat yoghurt
(approx. 350 calories)

Dinner: Homemade spaghetti Bolognese using 125 g of extra lean beef, 50 g of whole wheat spaghetti (dry weight), 200 g of chopped fresh tomatoes and unlimited optional ingredients such as carrots, onions, mushrooms, garlic etc. If you need to fry anything, use a one-cal cooking spray
(approx. 400 calories)

Snack 1: 1 medium glass of wine 175 ml,
(approx. 140 calories)

Snack 2/pudding: 2 fingers of Kit Kat
(approx. 110 calories)

8
MONITOR YOUR FAT INTAKE

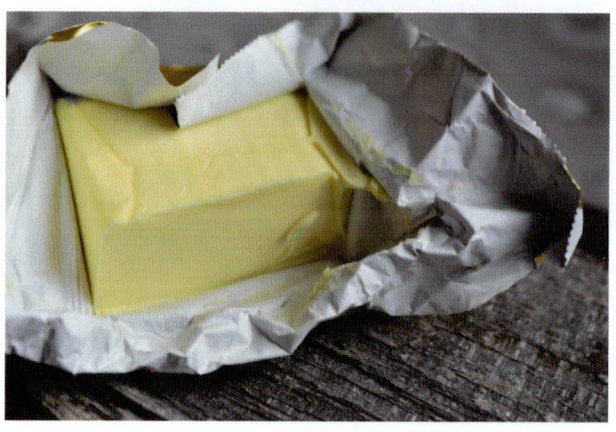

Here's what you need to know about fat: although fat has a bad reputation, it doesn't have to be the enemy. What matters is the type of fat you're eating and how much of it.

Your body needs fat to function properly. Fat is one of three essential macronutrients (along with carbohydrate and protein) and an important source of energy.

Our cells need it to function properly and it enables the body to absorb vitamins. It's also key to keeping our skin and hair healthy. The health risks of eating too much fat are associated with the consumption of unhealthy, saturated fats commonly found in fast foods, processed foods, refined foods, and animal products like meat (the type of foods people in the Western world tend to find appealing).

Saturated fat is calorie dense and therefore too much of it can lead to weight gain. Being overweight, as we know, can lead to serious life-threatening conditions such as Type 2 diabetes, heart disease , etc. The added issue with too much fat is that it can cause other problems (that aren't necessarily a result of just being overweight) such as high blood pressure, high cholesterol and gastrointestinal conditions such as colorectal and colon cancer.

In turn, some of those conditions can lead to other serious conditions such as stroke and heart attack.

So, if you are trying to lose weight and stay healthy, keep saturated fat consumption to a minimum.

Luckily, not all fats are created equal. Some fats are healthy – notably unsaturated fats found in oily fish, olive oil, nuts and seeds including peanut butter, some vegetables and fatty plant products e.g. coconut.

The main benefit of unsaturated fat is heart health. Unsaturated fat is known to lower the level of bad cholesterol in your blood (LDL) and elevate the level of good cholesterol in your blood (HDL). This is likely to reduce your chances of getting heart disease are.

So, go ahead, eat unsaturated fat, but don't overdo it. The Government recommends no more than 30 g per day for a man and 20 g daily for a woman.

There is another category of fat that you should avoid over all others because it can quickly increase the bad cholesterol in your blood if consumed regularly. It's called Trans Fat. Trans Fats are contained in hydrogenated oils primarily found in processed products such as cakes, biscuits, doughnuts, crisps, pies, pizza, fried food, non-dairy creamer, and some margarines.

Many companies no longer use Trans Fats, and the World Health Organisation has recommended that they're eliminated from all manufactured food from 2023.

9
KEEP PROPERLY HYDRATED

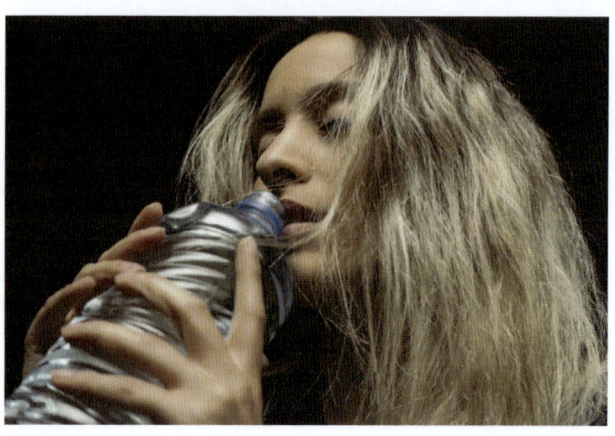

The body is made up of around 60% water. Water plays a huge role in many of the body's functions, so it's important to keep that level topped up by ensuring you take in enough liquid. Most of the time you can stay properly hydrated by listening to your body. When you're thirsty, drink something and if it's hot or you've been doing physical activity, drink more than usual.

Most guidance suggests you should be drinking at least 1.5 litres a day – which is good advice if you can manage it. Carry around a bottle with you to make that target easier to reach. But if water's not your thing, remember that much of the water we consume comes from the foods we eat. Also, liquids in general count, so remember to include tea, coffee, carbonated drinks etc.

You'll know if you're dehydrated because your urine will be dark yellow, Other signs and symptoms include constipation, headaches, dizziness, confusion and a dry mouth.

As we age, it's even more important to keep hydrated because our bodies retain less water, and the signs of dehydration are milder. Serious cases of dehydration can lead to death.

10

READ FOOD LABELS AND BE AWARE OF PORTION DISTORTION

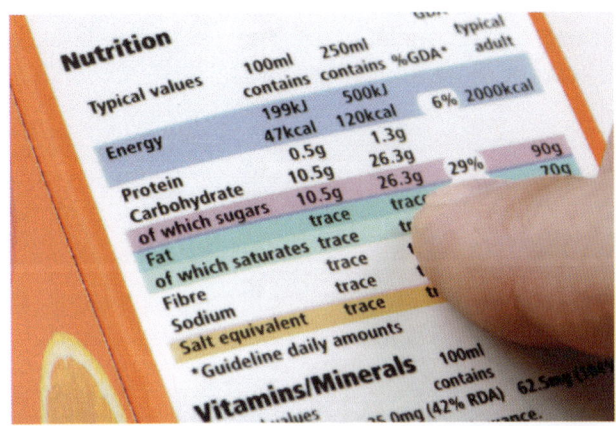

Every pre-packaged product is required to display ingredients and nutritional information. Read the labels and do your best to understand them, because once you've mastered the practice, eating healthily and within a calorie ceiling is a lot easier.

First, start with the **ingredients**, Labels show ingredients in descending order of weight, so if, sugar is one of the main ingredients of, say, a savoury ready meal, it's probably not a great choice.

Then have a look at the colours on the **'traffic light system'** label which tell you about the level of overall fats, saturated fats, sugar, and salt. Red is a high level, amber is a medium level and green is a low level. So, if at first glance most of the sections are coloured green, you can be fairly sure the product is healthy.

Calories are also displayed, but this is where it can get complicated because the devil is in the detail of how they are presented in terms of a 'serving size'. You might assume a serving size is the entire packet of something because the packet looks small to you. But the manufacturer may have decided that a serving size is just a third of the packet, in which case you would need to triple the calories if you wanted to eat it all. The other part of the label that can be confusing is the **'Typical Values'** area. This lists amounts for energy (calories), fat, carbohydrate, fibre, protein, and salt. The trouble with this section is that it's normally presented in the form of 'per 100 g', in which case you need to look at the total weight of the product, work out how much you estimate you would eat, then do a mathematical calculation to determine if the product's for you.

If it sounds like hard work, that's because it is, and it's quite possible to spend hours in a supermarket poring over labels while doing calculations. Some manufacturers make labels easier to read than others, but my advice is to get to grip with reading food labels through practice and if you're short of time or can't be bothered, just look at the traffic light system and make sure there's more green than red.

11

BEWARE: NOT ALL HEALTHY FOODS WILL HELP YOU LOSE WEIGHT

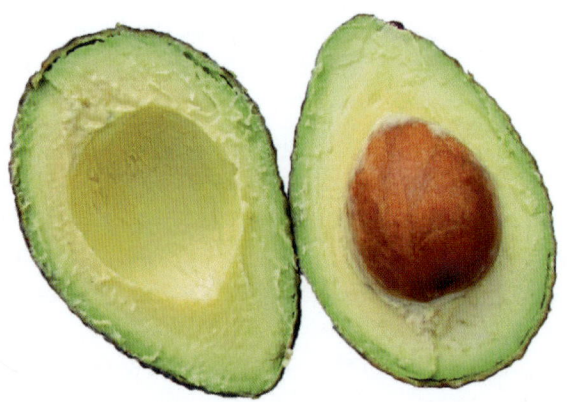

Take the fruit of the moment – avocados. They're considered healthy because they contain vitamins, minerals and heart-healthy unsaturated fat. They're low in carbs, high in fibre and contain antioxidants. They also taste nice. What's not to like?

Well, if you're trying to lose weight, quite a lot actually. An average avocado contains a startling 350 calories which is equivalent to the calorie counted lunch example I gave earlier. It's also made up of a whopping 77% fat. Although the fat is unsaturated and that's good for your heart, your body doesn't distinguish between saturated and unsaturated fat and if you don't burn it off through activity, it will be stored internally. Too much visceral fat (as it's known) around your internal organs is a bad thing because it can adversely affect the organ's efficiency.

Other healthy foods that you may consider avoiding in bulk for the same reason if you're trying to lose weight include nuts, seeds, olive oil, peanut butter, salmon, mackerel, dark chocolate, most coconut products, rib eye steak, whole milk, Greek yoghurt, hummus, fruit juices, dates, sports drinks, most cereal bars and many healthy ready meals — including veggie/vegan ones.

12

EAT SMART: SWAP REGULAR FOOD PRODUCTS FOR THEIR EQUIVALENT

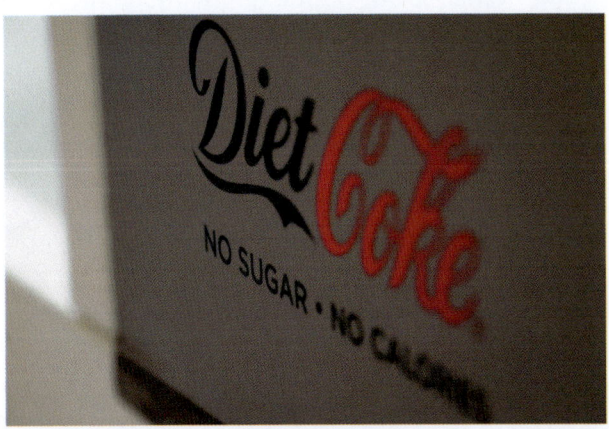

For many food and drink items sold in shops nowadays, there is an alternative for people who are watching their weight. Buy them, eat/drink them and grow to love them because they are extremely effective slimming tools. One of the most popular and successful of all time is the iconic drink Diet Coke which has zero calories compared to the original's 140 for a 330 ml can.

Look out for labels that say things like: 'DIET', 'LIGHT', 'SKINNY', 'LOW CALORIE', 'SLIMLINE', 'FAT FREE', 'L0-SUGAR', etc. Be careful though. If they sound too good to be true, they probably are — for example, you might buy a low-fat yoghurt thinking you are being virtuous, only to discover that the manufacturer has replaced the fat with extra sugar to give it taste.

Some of the most useful products include:

- Zero-calorie sweetener instead of sugar
- Low fat spread instead of butter
- Skimmed milk instead of full fat milk
- 1-cal cooking spray instead of cooking oil
- No-added-sugar soft drinks (including slimline ones as alcoholic mixers)
- Reduced fat meats e.g. minced beef
- Sauces including mayonnaise and tomato ketchup
- Cereals/cereal bars

Also, reduced calorie/fat/sugar versions of popular snacks such as crisps, biscuits, cakes, sweets, chocolate, cheese, popcorn, ice cream, ready meals, soups, baked beans, and hot chocolate mix.

A word of warning though. Many of these products are highly processed and packed with artificial ingredients including chemicals, flavourings, and e-numbers.

Aspartame, for example is the world's most popular sugar replacement sweetener and is found in more than 6,000 products. It sells well because it is cheap, doesn't leave the aftertaste of some of its competitors and is easily available. But some studies have linked it to serious diseases such as cancer, stroke, and dementia, as well as other ailments including headaches, mood disorders and intestinal problems. So, when making your swaps, think carefully.

13

EAT MORE - NOT LESS - FOOD

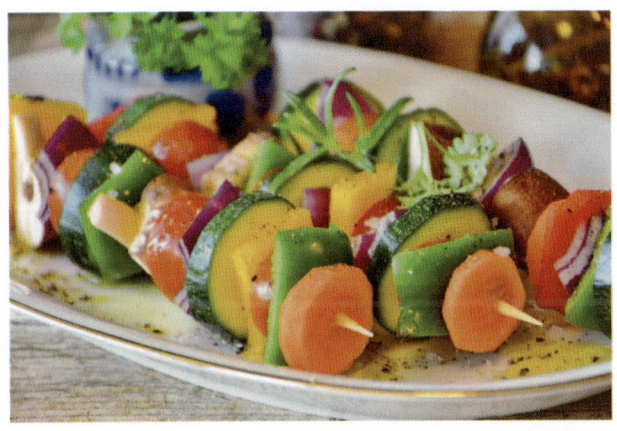

Many people believe that if you're trying to lose weight, the less food you eat the better. Dieters often miss meals in the mistaken assumption that fewer calories must lead to more weight loss.

Some people take it to extremes and develop an eating disorder in which they deny themselves food to such an extent they can't function properly.

Others with a severe eating disorder quite literally starve themselves to death.

Calories-in versus calories-out relates to the calorie deficit discussed previously and, yes, it is required to lose weight (although don't forget 'calories out' relates to exercise as well). But your body is a well-oiled machine and if you cut out too much food/calories it reacts accordingly by going into 'starvation mode' — i.e., it panics because it thinks survival is at stake. It then slows down your metabolism to preserve what food stores it has, and calorie output is reduced. In weight loss terms this means you're likely to plateau or even gain weight.

The process doesn't happen overnight, but reducing calories to super-low levels on a regular basis means you end up having to eat less…and then even less…and later on, much, much less to lose any weight whatsoever. To get caught in this cycle is physically and psychologically harmful.

So, one of the keys to losing weight is to eat sufficient food so that your metabolism chugs along happily promoting weight loss to the best of its ability.

Load up your plate with lots of healthy, calorie conscious food so that you feel satisfied after you've eaten. **Think about what foods you can add to your diet, rather than what foods you can remove.**

For example, if one of your favourite meals is battered fish, chips, mushy peas, and lashings of ketchup, you know it wouldn't be sensible to have it if you're trying to lose weight. You could, of course, have a couple of mouthfuls of the fish, four greasy chips and a dessertspoon of mushy peas to keep within a self-imposed calorie level, but that wouldn't be a meal — it would barely be a snack. In addition, the food would only cover a tiny area on your plate and you'd soon be hungry again. What should you do? I suggest something along these lines:

Substitute the fried fish with a salmon fillet, bake a potato (even better a sweet potato) and load up your plate with vegetables or salad - or both. If you want sauce, squirt a bit from a low calorie/low sugar ketchup or similar.

And then ENJOY! It might not be 'real' fish and chips, but it'll taste great, you'll have a big, satiating plate of food and you'll feel good because *you* made a pro-active sensible choice rather than a sacrifice. Do this sort of thing on a regular basis and you'll re-train your taste buds, re-educate your thought processes and satisfy your food urges in healthier ways.

14

SUPERFOODS – SUPER OR A SUPER SELLING STRATEGY?

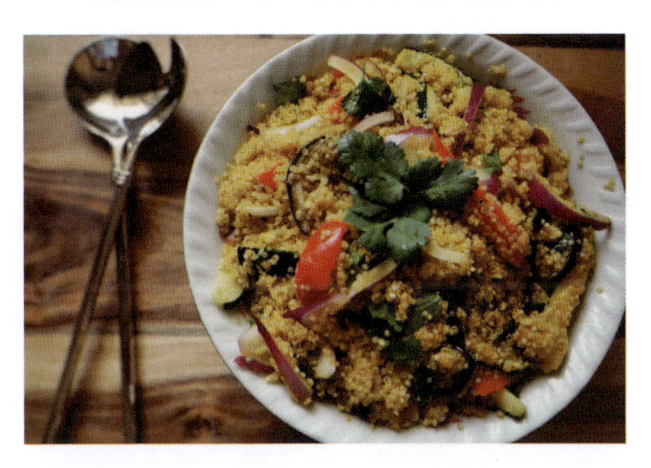

Let's be clear, there's NO such thing as a superfood. It's a trendy term invented by the marketing industry to sell products which are often super-expensive.

That's not to say there aren't some foods that are extremely healthy because they're nutritionally balanced and packed full of vitamins, minerals, essential fatty acids, amino acids, protein and antioxidants — some of the key components of 'superfoods'.

But have you noticed that superfoods are often lauded by celebrities who love to extol the virtues of ones we've never heard of? For example, are you familiar with amaranth, camu camu fruit, umeboshi and moringa? No, neither was I until I scrolled through Instagram and discovered them under the #celebritysuperfoods.

Most experts including doctors will tell you there are no miracle foods, and foods cannot cure incurable diseases (another claim of some superfoods) But, if there was, it would be…wait for it: **MILK.** That's because milk contains all the things (and more) that superfoods generally contain as well as calcium which is crucial for your bones as you age.

Milk is a staple of most people's fridges, it's cheap, has multiple uses and it's palatable — unlike some superfoods (have you ever had a plate of steamed kale!?)

So, drink milk if you want to tell people you're into superfoods, only make it semi-skimmed or skimmed for maximum health benefits.

And do you realise that foods which have been around since the beginning of time have now been promoted to superfood status? Examples include berries, avocado, quinoa, broccoli, kale, spinach, oats, turmeric, garlic, seeds, nuts and tea variations including green and matcha.

15

TO PROTEIN SUPPLEMENT OR NOT TO SUPPLEMENT, THAT IS THE QUESTION?

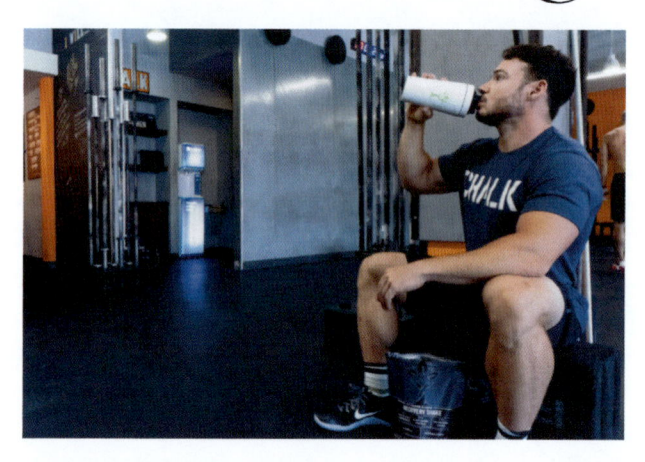

And the answer is? Probably not. When the term supplement is used in connection with food and diet nowadays, people are normally referring to protein supplements.

You've seen the super-exercisers at the gym parading around with their protein shakes in plastic bottles. And you've been into shops and seen row after row of protein bars and those huge tubs of powder that you know have something to do with bigger muscles, but you're not quite sure what.

What you do know, though, is that these products are incredibly expensive and even though you can't afford them, you can't help wondering whether you're missing out because they must work as the rest of the world seems to be taking them.

Let's get something straight, unless you're a full-on body builder or athlete you don't *need* to protein supplement. **An average woman needs around 45-50 g a day and an average man needs around 55-60 g a day.** This level can easily be derived from the food you eat in a healthy, balanced diet. However, it is true to say that when you are exercising intensely and trying to increase your muscle mass, your protein requirements increase. To calculate your needs if you fall into this category, **multiply your body weight in kgs by 1.2 g if you're an average woman and by 1.4 g if you're a man.**

For example, a woman weighing 60 kg and working out regularly and intensely (including lifting weights) would need 60 X 1.2 = 72 g per day.

At this level, it can be tricky to incorporate enough protein into your diet. In these circumstances, a protein supplement would be helpful. It is, after all, convenient and you don't have to load up your plate with food sources of protein that, under normal circumstances, you wouldn't choose to eat.

But beware, just because it's a protein supplement and you bought it from a health food shop, doesn't mean it's good for you in other ways. Look for the ingredients that you might not expect to feature heavily - such as sugar - by reading the labels. Many protein supplements are very calorific which is fine if you're a body builder trying to bulk-up, but far from fine if you're someone trying to lose weight as well as build muscle.

16

EAT - DON'T DRINK – YOUR FRUIT

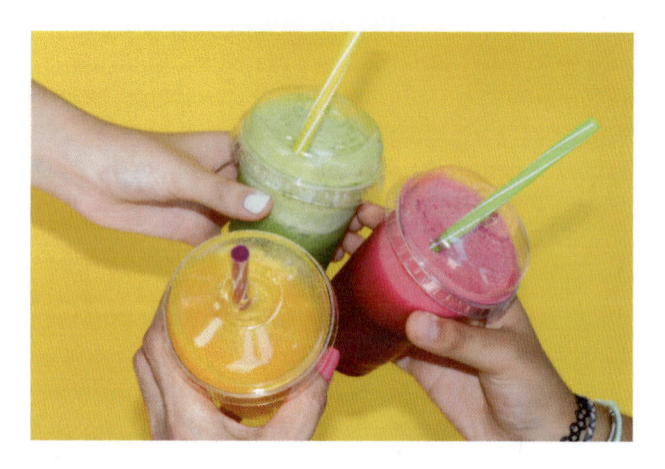

It's on-trend to juice, and fruit smoothies taste great. In that regard there's nothing wrong with them…but you would be far better off eating the whole fruit.

That's because fruit is packed with sugar — natural sugar yes, but sugar all the same which, as we know, is not good for your health and is calorific.

The trouble with fruit smoothies is that you need to put quite a lot of fruit into the blender in order to make a decent sized drink.

The situation worsens when you buy a pre-packaged smoothie from a shop or order one in a restaurant because they often contain 'hidden' additives to make them taste nicer: such as yoghurt, ice cream or whole milk.

Also, because you drink rather than eat a smoothie, your body absorbs the sugar a lot more rapidly. This will initially lead to a blood sugar spike, but later a low. This sort of change messes with your insulin levels which can cause longer term problems. The worst of it is, if your body doesn't use the sugar for energy, it WILL be stored as fat.

But there are other reasons why smoothies aren't as healthy as they seem — agitation in the blender during the juicing process bashes the life out of the fruits' fibre and therefore decreases their effectiveness. Also, smoothies don't satiate you in the same way as whole food does. So, you'll get hungrier sooner and may end up eating more than you planned.

The answer? If you love your fruit, eat it whole and if you love smoothies, make them with vegetables — it's hard to make an unhealthy veggie smoothie.

It would be unwise for a book like this not to explore diets that once started as fads or trends but are now firmly established in popular diet and lifestyle culture. The reason for this is that they actually work for many people — a statement backed up by studies. I am, of course, talking about **intermittent fasting, keto, clean eating, and veganism.**

17
TRY DIET TYPES THAT HAVE BEEN PROVEN TO WORK FOR OTHERS

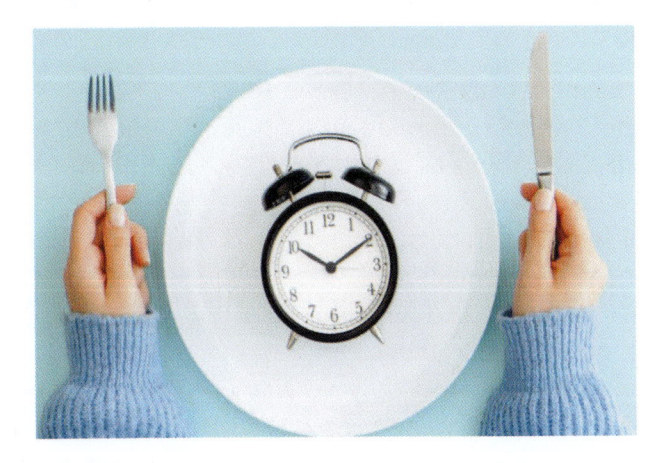

There's a lot a hype and hyperbole surrounding these very diverse diets, but what they all have in common is a premise that they contribute to a healthy lifestyle. Most aid weight loss too.

Here's an explanation of what each one is, and its benefits, to help you decide if you want to try one.

INTERMITTENT FASTING (IF)

A slightly confusing term because you don't fast, as such, you just eat the meals you're having within a restricted time frame. There are several different IF methods, one of the most popular is delaying your first meal of the day until midday and having your next around 8pm. This means you're not eating for approximately 16 hours, including the time when you're asleep. It also means you're skipping one of your three meals a day. Unsurprisingly this can lead to weight loss. Research also shows IF can improve your metabolic health (the efficient chemical processes in cells) protect against disease and help you live longer.

KETO

(Short for ketogenic): the keto diet involves drastically reducing carbs and replacing them with fats. The idea is that you put your body into a metabolic state called **ketosis** during which it becomes incredibly efficient at burning fat for energy. This is because there's not enough carbohydrate (the body's first choice for fuel) to do the job. The knock-on effect is a reduction in blood sugar and insulin levels which means people with Type 2 Diabetes can benefit. Weight loss on a keto diet is common.

CLEAN EATING

Eating clean means restricting your consumption to unprocessed, whole, nutrient-dense foods as close to their natural state as possible. So, lots of wholegrain foods, fruit, nuts, seeds, lean meats, and dairy products such as milk, natural yogurt, etc. Organic foods mainly come under the clean eating banner, partly because they've not been sprayed with synthetic pesticides, or are genetically engineered.

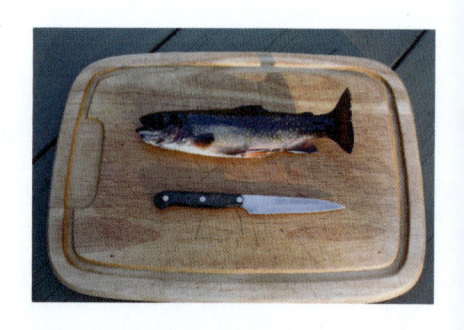

Clean eating means avoiding refined foods such as white bread, pasta, rice etc or refined sugars, junk or fried food (and if you buy pre-packaged foods the fewer ingredients on the label, the better). Clean eating reduces inflammation in the body – the cause of many modern-day diseases and boosts the immune system. It can increase your energy levels, prevent gut and digestive problems, and help you lose weight.

VEGAN

If you're vegan you eat no animal products whatsoever. You diet is derived from plants - particularly vegetables, fruits, grains, nuts, and pulses.

That's it, other than to say veganism is often more than just a diet, it's a belief system. Vegans do what they can to develop a world in which no animal is harmed in service to humans. Eating no animal products can be an extremely healthy way of living and it can help with weight loss. However, care is needed to ensure your diet includes all the essential nutrients often found in animal products such as protein, vitamin B12, iron and omega 3 fatty acids (contained in things like oily fish).

18

MONITOR YOUR PROGRESS, RECORD RESULTS & IF NECESSARY, SET NEW GOALS

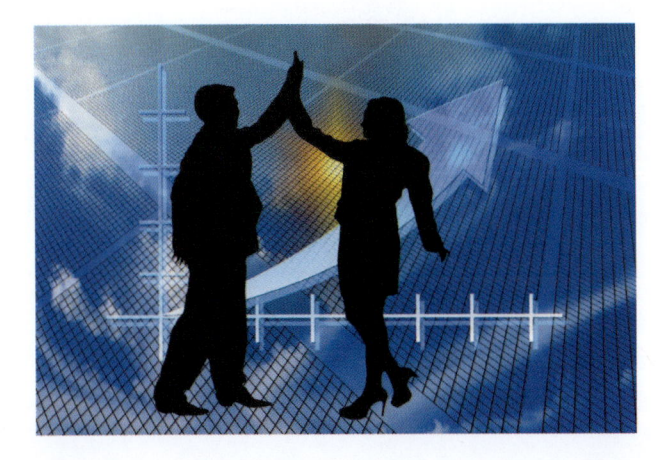

Decide in advance how often you are going to measure your progress and stick to it – even if you've had a bad day/week/month. I do not recommend you weigh yourself more than once week though. The reason for this is that the body fluctuates on a day-to-day basis due to many transient factors such as menstruation, dehydration, water retention, a heavy meal the night before, constipation, exercise, salty food, or a lot of caffeine. Over seven days these things tend to balance out.

The best, and most accurate time to weigh yourself is after you get up and before you've had anything to eat or drink. To make accurate comparisons, stick to the same day, time and *location every time you jump on the scales, so you can compare like with like. This also goes for what clothes (if any)/jewellery/shoes etc you are wearing.

*scales should be used on a hard floor rather than carpet.

PART TWO

EXERCISE

This next section focuses on exercise – why you should do it, what to do, how to do it and ways to make it effective, enjoyable, and sustainable.

Exercise works in many ways, but the right type done in the right way, addresses the issues of being fat and unfit at the same time.

That's because exercise burns calories and fat – the metabolic process required to create the weight loss catalyst, calorie deficit.

Exercise also enables your body to work a lot more efficiently, particularly your heart – which is significant in terms of a longer life, less disease, and your ability to fight disease.

It also benefits that all-important organ - the brain - and therefore your mental health (more on that in Part 3).

In the early stages of the COVID-19 pandemic in 2020, the Government's chief medical officer, Professor Chris Whitty, couldn't have made the importance of exercise any clearer. He said:

> "There is no situation, there is no age and no condition where exercise is not a good thing"

During another speech he added:

> "Exercise is central to a happy and healthy old age"

CASE STUDY 1
Viv, 52

Before we go into the details of exercise, let's meet our first case study, Viv, whose life was transformed through exercise.

Mother of two, Viv, worked in the fine art licensing business for many years before giving up her job to care full time for her daughter who has a severe disability. The new role took its toll but during her 40s Viv was able to cope with the stress, sleep deprivation and physical exertion that was part of her new lifestyle. She self-medicated with wine, convenience foods and the odd jog in the park and she thought she was fine…until one day she wasn't.

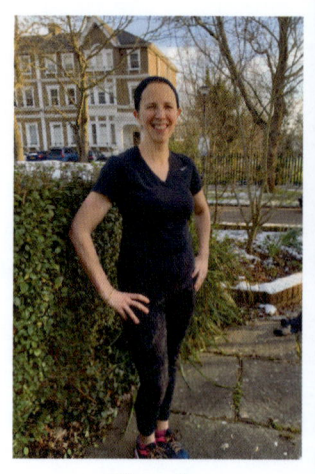

Viv today

A trip to the GP revealed her blood pressure was through the roof. She was prescribed high dosage medication to regulate it, although her doctor suggested she might have to accept hypertension as a 'disease of old age'.

She had also developed psoriasis which was getting worse with time. Now in her late 40's Viv was entering perimenopause which brought a whole new set of problems including weight gain. The trouble was, she hadn't realised what was causing them and certainly hadn't made the hormonal link to why she was so tense, emotional and irritable. On top of that, her self-esteem plummeted and she lost confidence in her body — how it looked and what it could do. She was at a low point in her life, a crossroads, and although she didn't know it at the time, exercise was to be her saviour. Viv decided to join her local gym. At first she just enjoyed the time-out and the headspace the trips there gave her. She did a bit of gentle running and cycling before realising it wasn't going to be enough to make much difference. So, she hired a personal trainer – ME!

> *"Getting a PT was one of the best decisions I have ever made and the effects have been far reaching. My primary goal was simply to look a bit trimmer and be physically stronger for my caring role. If I could lower my blood pressure too - something I had thought was going to be impossible — it would be an amazing bonus."*

"Over the months I transformed physically and mentally. After a year, my blood pressure moved from hyper to pre-hypertensive; then to normal and is now in the 'optimum' level range. I have lost 10 kg in weight and have gone from a B.M.I of 24.6 to a B.M.I of 20.7. And, I'm pleased to say that much of the weight has gone from around my middle which is quite an achievement for someone like me who has an 'apple' shaped body."

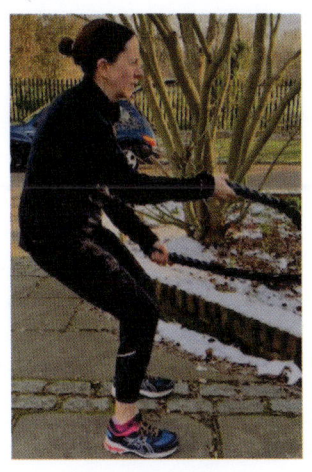

Viv doing heavy resistance work

Viv, who also runs a charity for carers, continued:

"Another unexpected benefit has been the calming of my psoriasis. I enjoy telling surprised medics that exercise has been effective treatment where steroids have failed. I love my new strength which keeps me able to meet the physical challenges of caring. I see people of my age struggling to get out of a chair, while I can do press ups, burpees, crunches, and heavy resistance work as well as run 5K in 35 minutes. I also love the physical manifestation of it — defined muscles in my arms and legs which means I no longer worry about uncovering in the summer."

She continued:

"The new strength is not just physical though. I have a different mindset which enables me to compartmentalise the challenges I have but, perhaps more importantly, enables me to be comfortable with not being comfortable."

Viv also changed her diet but didn't 'go on a diet.' Out went convenience foods and in came healthy home-cooked versions of them with a focus on smaller portions, low G.I foods (foods that are broken down slowly by the body), plenty of fruit and veg and much less meat. She said:

"I don't stress over food now because I see it as a source of fuel for my exercise. I love heathy fats and treats. Wine is one of them, but it's become an end-of-week treat rather than a daily anaesthetic.

She concluded:

> *"These small individual changes in fitness, diet, strength and mental health, have had a knock-on cumulative effect that adds up to a profound impact. Thankfully, they came just in time to give me the toolkit and resilience required to get through the menopause without HRT.*
>
> *I now focus on all the things my body can do and I've been trying adventurous pursuits that I would never have considered before — like rock climbing.*
>
> *I feel like somebody gave me the key to the door and all I had to do was unlock it. That door's staying open from now on and I've thrown away the key!"*

An inspiring story, I hope you'll agree.

Now it's your turn to catch the exercise bug and you're going to need an action plan.

Before you start an exercise programme you should collect some base line fitness statistics so that you have something to compare your progress with later down the line.

19

DO A CARDIOVASCULAR FITNESS TEST

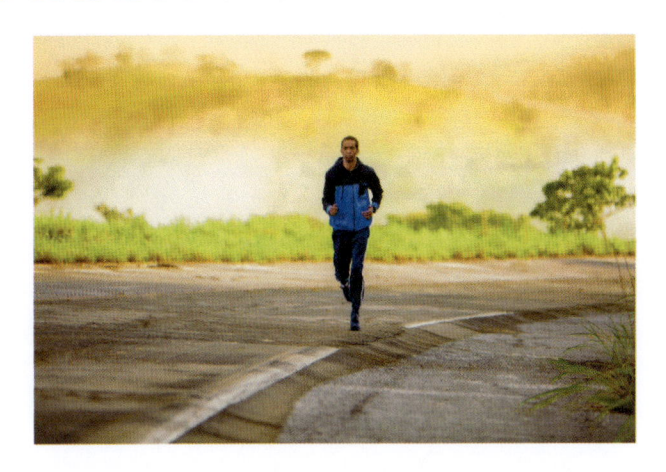

How far can you walk, jog or run in 12 minutes? (if you can run, you should do so; if you can jog, then do so; and if walking's your limit, that's fine).

How did you do?

Age 50+	Excellent	Above Average	Average	Below Average	Poor
Female	More than 2.2 km	1.7-2.2 km	1.4-1.7 km	1-1.4 km	Less than 1 km
Male	More than 2.4 km	2-2.4 km	1.6-2 km	1.3-1.6 km	Less than 1.3 km

20

DO A CORE STRENGTH TEST

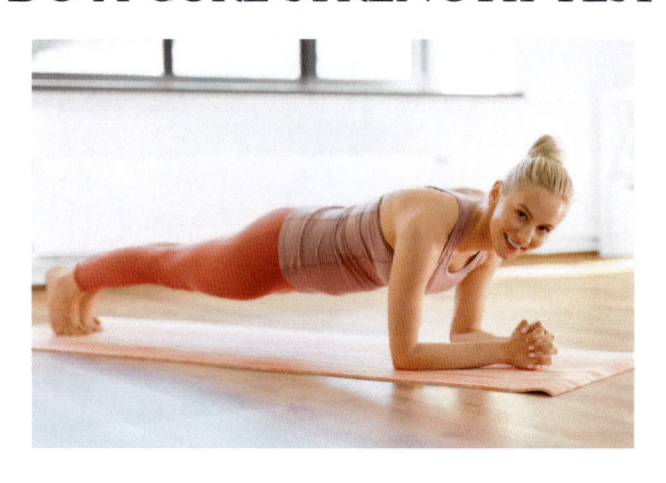

There are many different types of strength – explosive, endurance, relative, maximum and so on, but the key ones for beginners are core and upper body.

How long can you hold a low plank for?

Age 50+	Excellent	Very Good	Good	Average	Below Average	Poor
Female And Male	Over 3 mins	2-3 mins	1-2 mins	30-45 secs	20-30 secs	Below 20 secs

21

DO AN UPPER BODY STRENGTH TEST

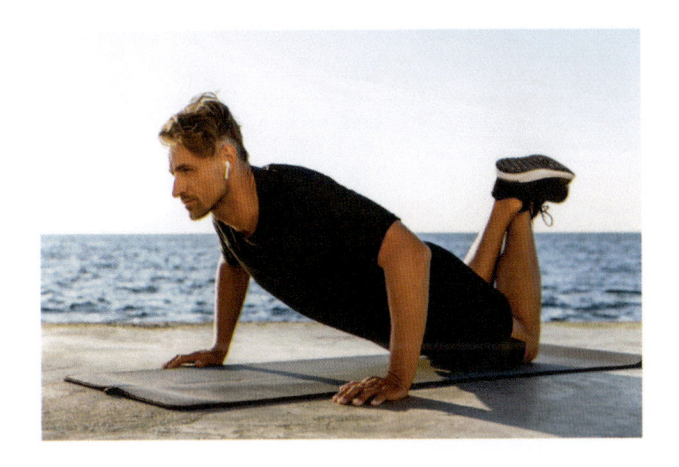

How many press ups on your knees can you do without stopping?

Technique: kneel on the floor, hands either side of your chest and underneath your shoulders. Keep your back straight. Bend elbows and lower yourself until your elbows are at right angles and your nose is nearly touching the floor. Push up, repeat.

Age 50+	Excellent	Very Good	Fair	Poor
Female And Male	More than 30	15-29	6-14	1-5

22

DO A FLEXIBILITY TEST:

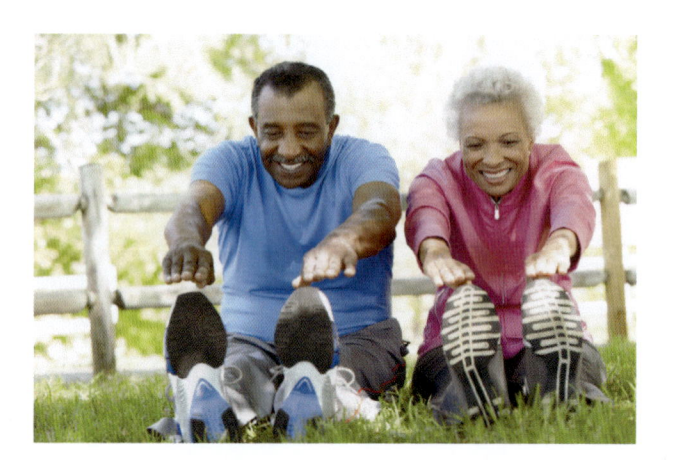

This test is known as the 'sit and reach' test. You need someone to help you with it.

Sit down with your legs straight out in front of you flat on the floor. With both hands, reach down for your toes and when you get to your furthest point, hold for a couple of seconds. The other person should now measure the distance the tips of your fingers are - either before your toes or, if you're more flexible, in front of your toes.

Age 50+	Excellent	Very Good	Good	Fair	Poor
Female And Male	More than 5 cm in front of your toes	Just in front of your toes	Toe level	Up to 5 cm before your toes	More than 5 cm before your toes

You should now have **8 starting statistics:** weight, BMI, body fat percentage, waist to hip ratio, cardio fitness, core strength, upper body strength and flexibility.

Why not compile a table with the dates and results of the tests and update it over time when you repeat the challenges. Keep it in a prominent place for motivation.

We now come to the exercise itself. For the purposes of this book we are going to **divide it into 6 categories:**

Cardio, resistance, abs and core, upper body strength, hips-thighs-glutes, and flexibility.

The rationale behind this is that if you choose exercises from each category for each of your training sessions you will get a full body workout which is my recommended format – whatever your age. And, depending on what your goals are, you can choose to omit a category or spend more time doing exercises from one category than another.

For each section I am going to list my top 5 exercises. It would be impossible to include every exercise in every category because the book would never end.

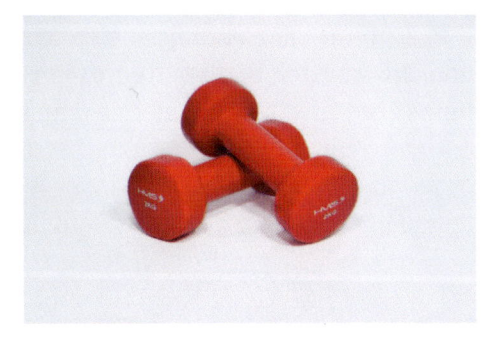

I have chosen the exercises because they can all be done from home as well as in a gym. Also, they're challenging but do-able for short periods of time for mature people. You can, of course, add your own exercises as you see fit. There are thousands of resources out there to help you do this both online and in print.

For each exercise listed, there will be a modified, easier option (apart from the stretches) and you only need equipment for the resistance and upper body section. If you have, or can purchase, dumbbells I recommend 2kg ones for beginner women and 3kg ones for beginner men. An alternative is two food cans of equal weight, two bags of sugar, or you could fill two plastic milk containers with water or sand.

But before any of that, you should…

23

LEARN HOW TO DO THE 'KING' AND 'QUEEN' OF ALL EXERCISES - SQUATS AND LUNGES

Squats and lunges are two vital building block exercises that work in similar ways to strengthen and condition all the major muscle groups of the lower body. That means the quadriceps (the front of the upper legs), the hamstrings (the back of the upper legs) and the glutes (the various muscles in your butt). The exercises also work your calves, your hips, your thighs, your lower back and your core. For beginners, squats are easier to do than lunges because less balance is required.

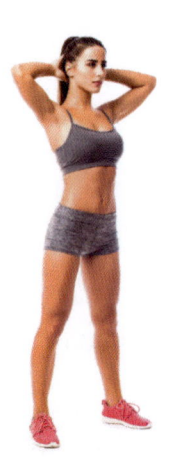

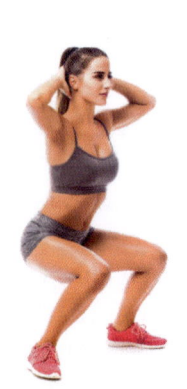

This is how to do a squat:
   Start standing with your feet shoulder width apart and you knees slightly outwards. Lower yourself as if you're sitting down on a tiny chair to the point where your hips are parallel to the ground. Once down, push back up through the heels to standing. During the downward phase make sure your knees are well back so that you can see the tip of your trainers. Keep your shoulders and chest back, and your head up.

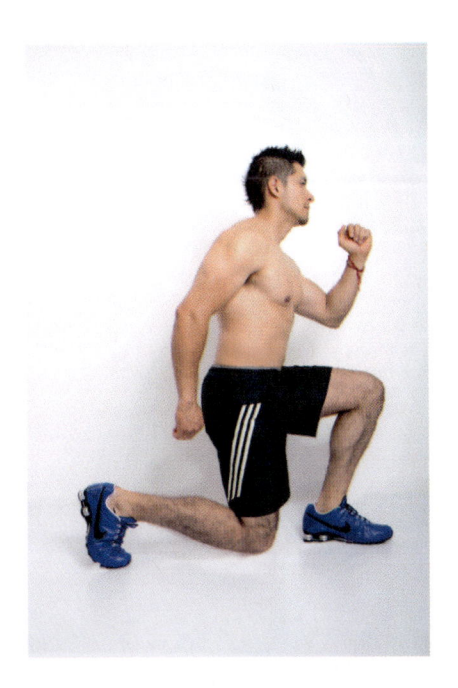

This is how to do a lunge:

Start upright and step forward with one foot until the knee at the front is at a 90-degree angle — as is the knee the back. Lift your front leg and return to the start position and do the same with the other leg going forward. Throughout the movement keep your torso upright and your shoulders back. Once the basic technique of squats and lunges has been mastered, you can try one of the numerous variations that exist (see resistance section).

24

DO CARDIO EXERCISES, INCLUDING THE FOLLOWING

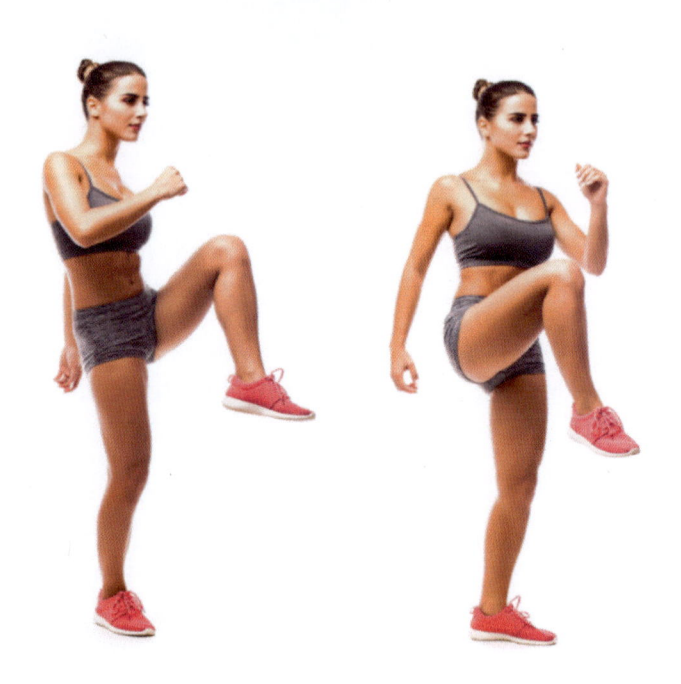

Jogging/running/high knees on the spot:
Lift and lower knees on the spot in a jogging rhythm. Move your arms backwards and forwards. To increase intensity, speed up the jog to a run and raise knees higher **(easier option: step up and down).**

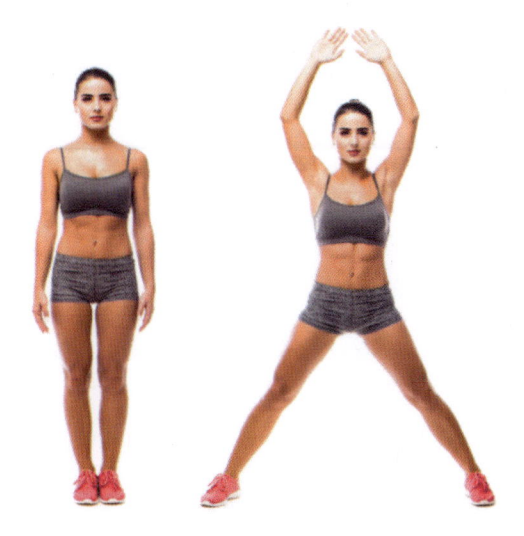

Jumping jacks:
Start with your feet near to each other, jump your feet wide with a slight bend of the knee and your arms reaching towards your head. Then reverse the process **(easier option: do one leg at a time).**

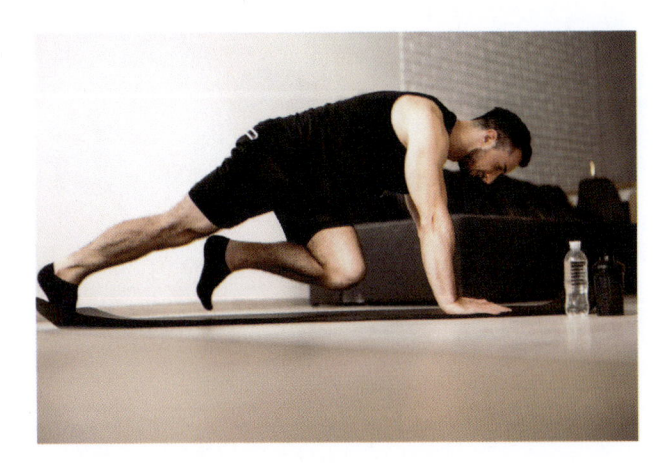

Mountain climbers:
Start in the push up position with your hands underneath your shoulders. Take one knee forward with the foot off the floor and then swap the legs over as if you're running in that position **(easier option: as the knee comes forward, tap the other toe and do it slowly).**

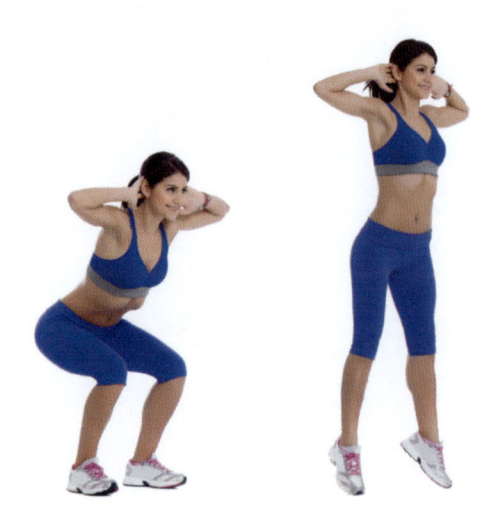

Squat jumps:
Stand tall with your feet shoulder width apart. Hinge backwards from the hips pushing your butt backwards so that your thighs are parallel to the ground, then launch yourself into a jump, land with bended knees at approximately 45 degrees then repeat **(easier option: leave out the jump, simply rise upwards on tip toes and return to the flat of the feet).**

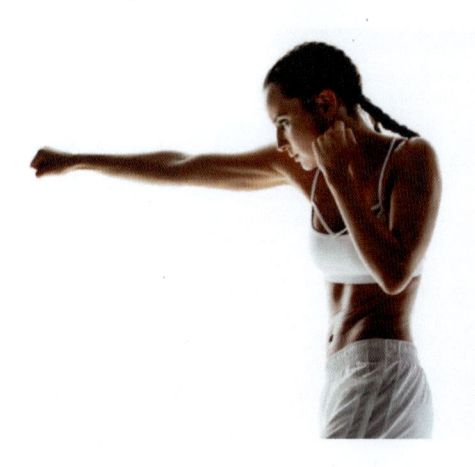

Side jog punch:
Start standing at an angle with knuckles clenched near the face. Jog forward with one leg and as you do so punch the same arm forward, then retreat to the starting position. Repeat in quick succession. Once you've done one side, switch to the other **(easier option: step and punch rather than jog).**

AS we age, we naturally lose muscle mass which can lead to weakness, instability, reduction of functionality and bone issues. Therefore, it is important for mature people to do resistance or strength training to build muscle to combat the change. It's an important element for weight loss too because muscle burns more calories than fat — even at rest.

25

DO SQUAT AND LUNGE EXERCISES WITH DUMBBELLS, INCLUDING THE FOLLOWING

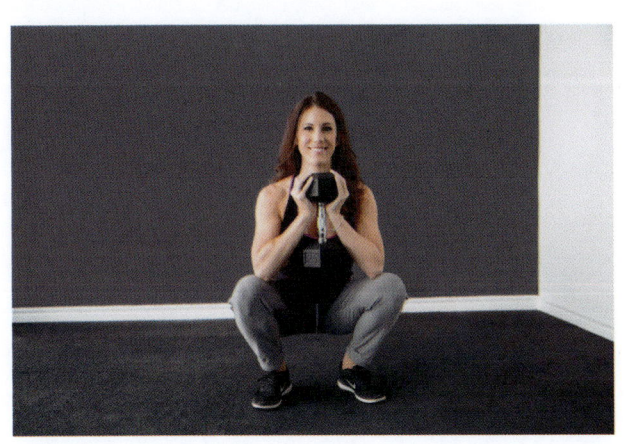

Goblet squat

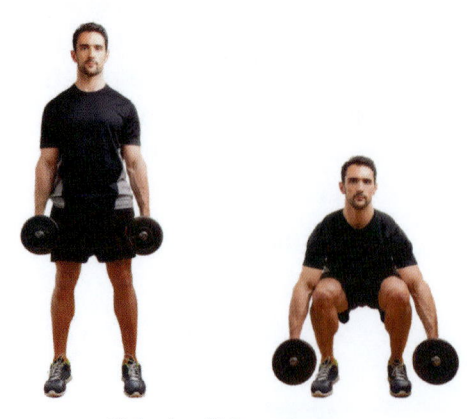

Side deadlift squat

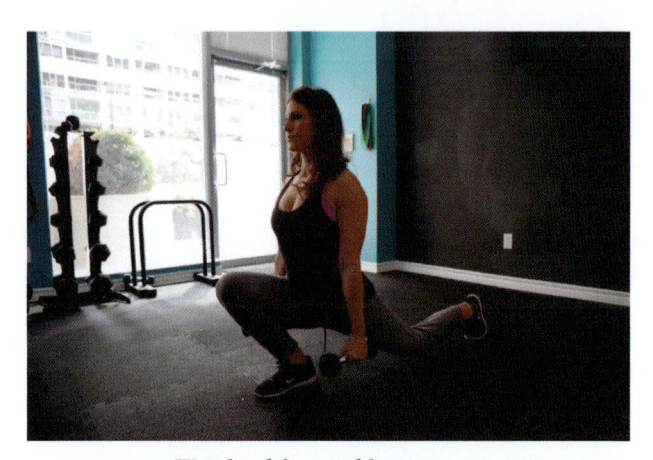

Weighted forward lunge

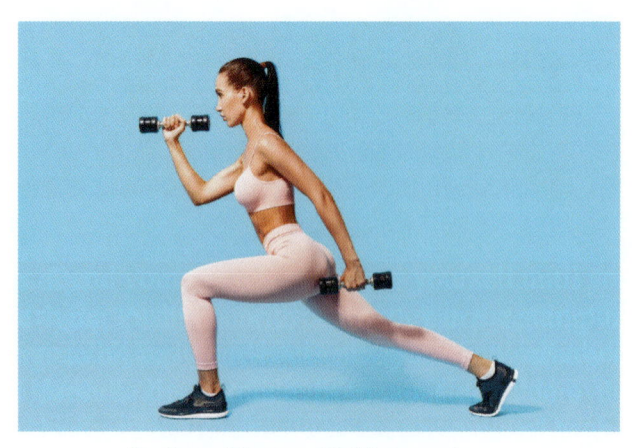

Backward lunge with bicep curl

Almost everybody who is trying to lose weight or who wants a 'better', healthier body, wants a flatter more toned stomach. The truth is: abs are made in the kitchen. This means if you're trying to get washboard abdominals, you first have to address the issue of the layer of fat covering your stomach and this is done primarily by reducing your calorie and fat intake.

The good news, however, is that everyone has a six pack lurking underneath their belly fat.

If you train your abdominal and core muscles at the same time as you're eating in a way designed to reduce your internal fat, then at some point you should start seeing definition which is the nearest thing an average person will get to a six pack.

26

DO ABDOMINAL AND CORE EXERCISES, INCLUDING THE FOLLOWING

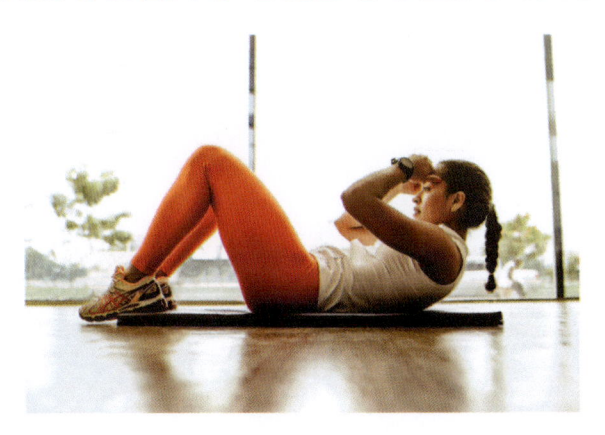

Basic crunches:
Lie on your back with your knees bent and your feet flat on the floor. Place your hands by your ears and raise your shoulders and chest off the ground. When you are about a third of the way up, lower head back to the floor and repeat **(easier option: place your hands on the front of your thighs and slide them up towards the knees as you crunch up and back down as you lower).**

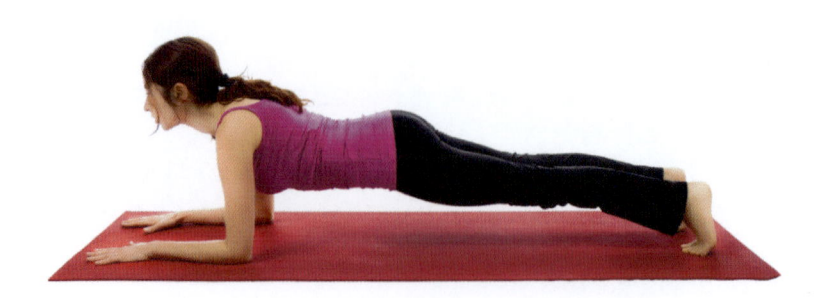

Plank hold:
Lie face down flat on the floor and using your forearms and toes push up into the plank position. Keep your back flat and your hips and butt down and in alignment. (see top pic, left) Brace your stomach muscles and hold for as long as possible. The world record is over 8 hours but if you can do a minute, that's a good start! **(easier option: push up with forearms but keep knees on the floor).**

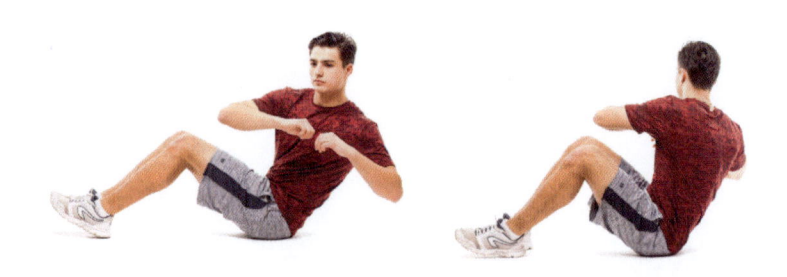

Russian twist:
Sit on the floor with your knees bent and your feet raised. Either with or without a weight, take both arms over to one side, then over to the other, pausing very briefly in the middle. The more you lean back, the harder it is. **(easier option: keep feet on the floor).**

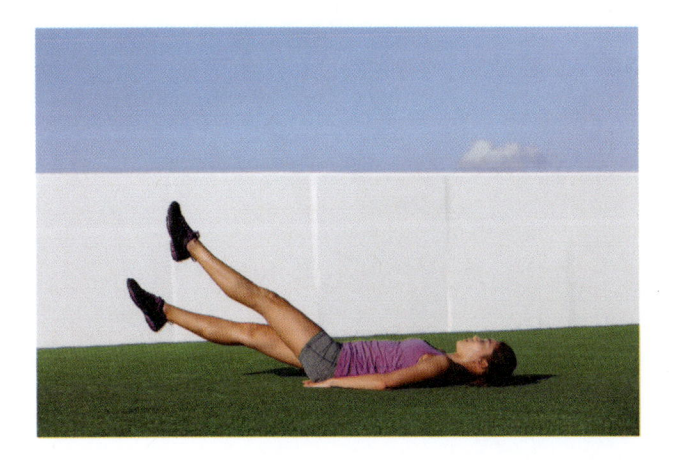

Flutter kicks:
Lie on your back with your shoulders off the floor and raise both your legs a few centimetres. Move one foot up and the other foot down in quick succession making sure you don't arch your back **(easier option: place your hands underneath your butt and place your head on the ground).**

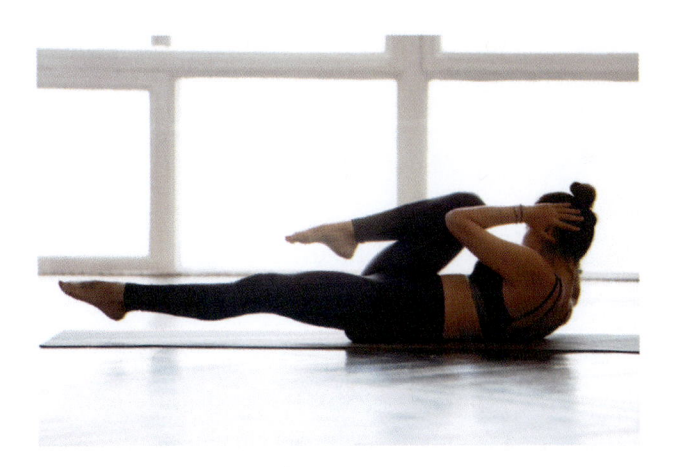

Bicycle crunches:
Lie on you back with your hands at the side of your head. Straighten your right leg out to a 45-degree angle while turning your upper body to the left. See if you can twist far enough so that you touch the opposite knee with your elbow. Do the same thing on the other side continuously either fast or slow **(easier option: just move the legs in and out 'locomotion' style).**

27
DO UPPER BODY STRENGTH EXERCISES, INCLUDING THE FOLLOWING

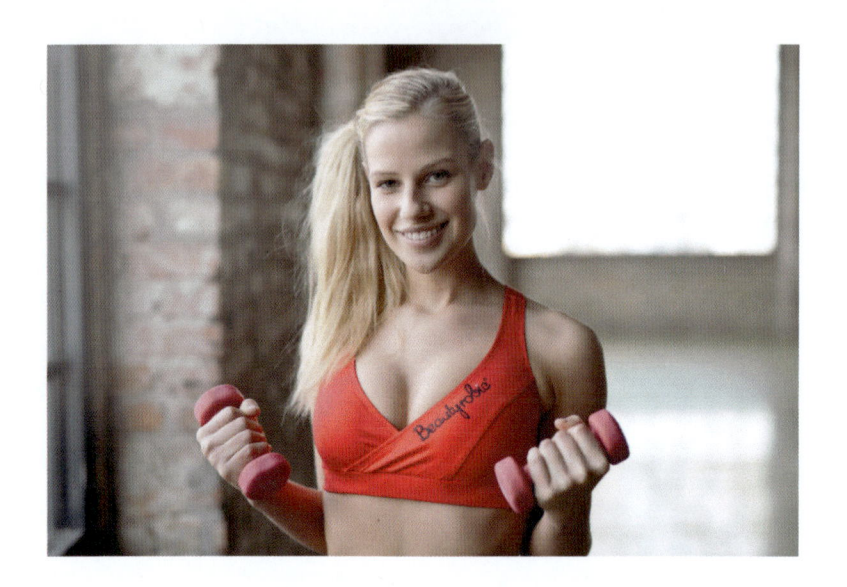

Bicep curls:
Hold two dumbbells with an underhand grip slightly wide of each thigh. Raise them up to your shoulders and lower them under control until your arms are extended. **(easier option: use a lighter weight, sit down while doing it or do one arm at a time).**

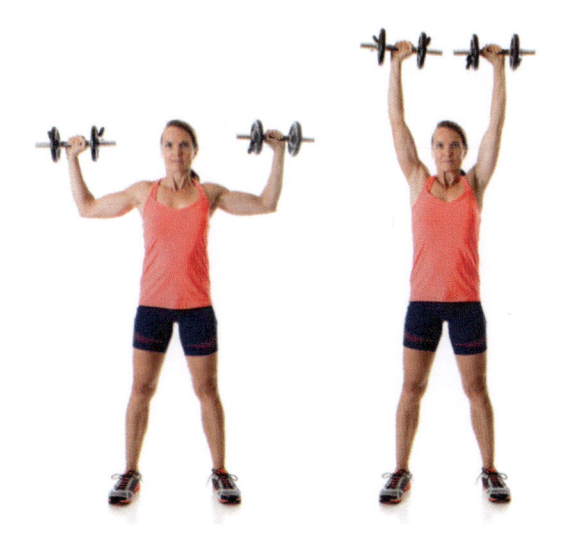

Overhead shoulder press:
Hold two dumbbells horizontally with an overhand grip at shoulder level, raise them upwards (and very slightly outwards) until they nearly meet at the top over your head. Return to start position and repeat. **(easier option; use a lighter weight, sit down while doing it or do one arm at a time).**

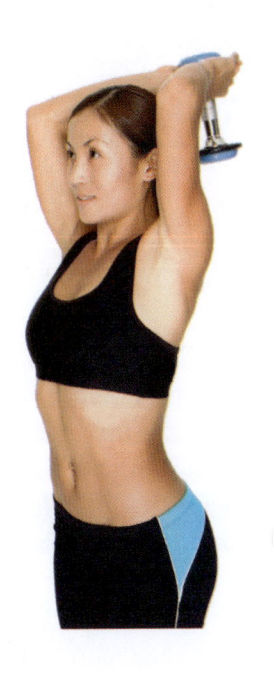

Tricep extension:
Stand tall with one dumbbell held over your head with straight arms. Flex your elbows and lower the weight down your back squeezing your shoulder blades together as you go. Keep your elbows as near to your ears as possible. Bring the weight back up the same way and tilt it upright when you get to the top. Do not come further forward than the front of the head. **(easier option: use no weight or sit down whilst doing it).**

Dumbbell Lateral raise:
Hold dumbbells at the side of your thighs and raise them outwards up to shoulder level. A slight bend of the arm is permissible. Lower them under control and repeat. **(easier option: use a lighter weight, sit down while doing it or do one arm at a time).**

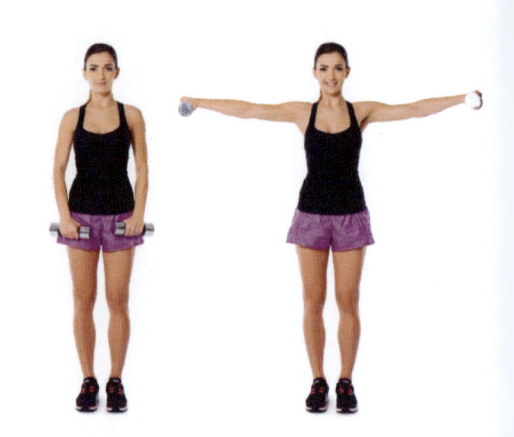

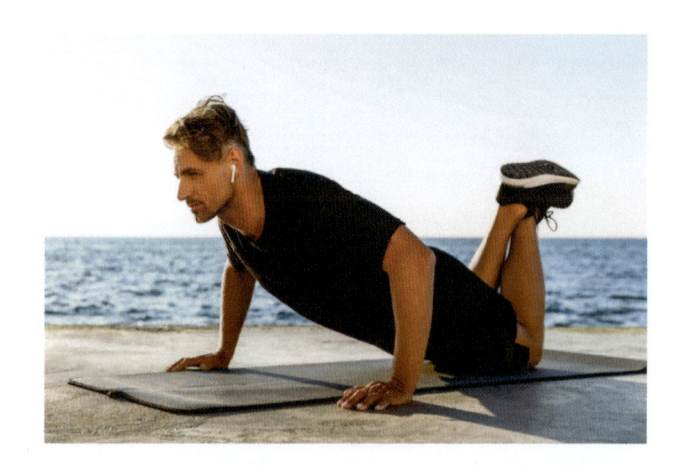

Press up/push up:
One of the oldest, hardest and most effective upper body exercises known to man. Start from an all-fours position with your hands slightly wider than shoulders. Push upwards so that your bodyweight is supported by your hands and toes. Bend your elbows and lower yourself until your elbows are at a 90 degree angle. Push up until you're back in the start position without locking your arms. Keep your back straight throughout **(easier option: drop to your knees to do it).**

Backside, booty, bum, rear, butt, buns, derriere, bottom…whatever you want to call it, the most fashionable part of your body to train right now (if you're a woman) is your glutes.

Glutes is the generic name for the various muscles in your posterior. If you only want a shapely behind, then look no further than the numerous variations of squats and lunges that exist – preferably with some form of resistance. Go into any gym and you'll see women doing just this – desperately trying to achieve a Kim Kardashian butt-look (see pic on right). However, if you want to train the whole area from below your abdomen to the bottom of your thighs, you have to work your glutes, your hips, your abductors (outer thighs) and your adductors (inner thighs). To do this:

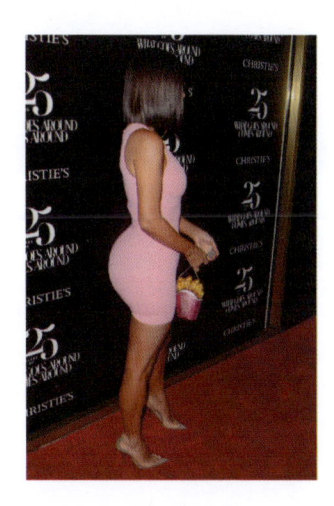

28

DO HIP, THIGH & GLUTE EXERCISES, INCLUDING THE FOLLOWING

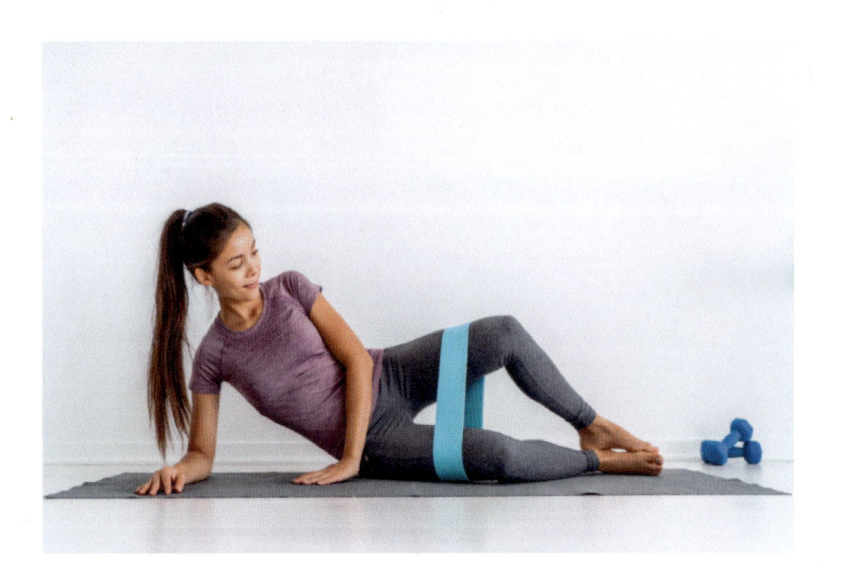

Clamshell:
Lie on your side and prop yourself up with one hand pressed against your ear. Draw your knees towards your chest. Keeping your feet in contact with each other, open and close the top leg 'clam'-style. For added intensity, wear a resistance band around your thighs.

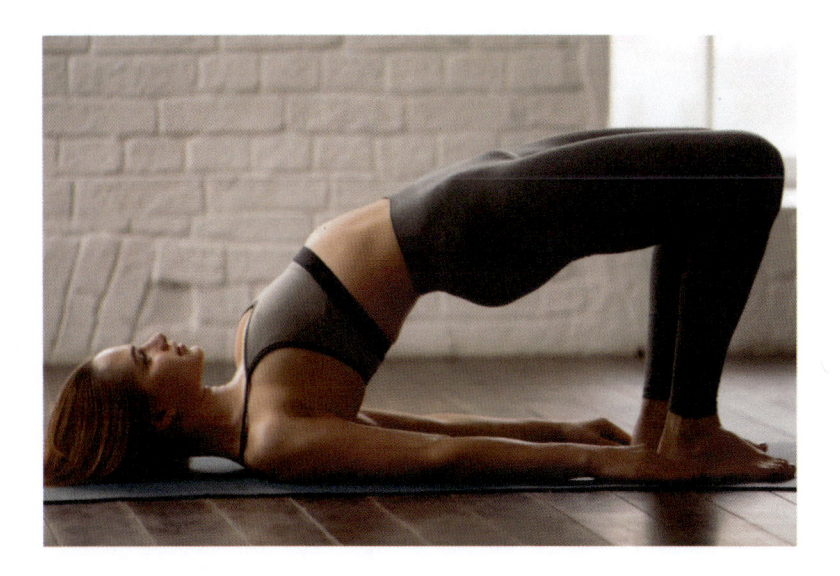

Glute bridge raise:
Lie on your back with your hands by your sides. Push hips and butt up as high as you can, then lower under control. Squeeze your glutes on the way up and relax them on the way down **(easier option: raise hips and butt halfway up).**

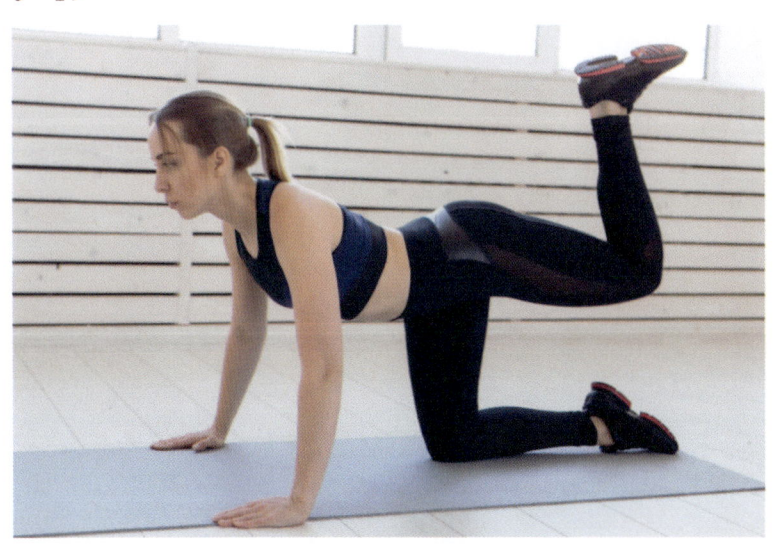

Donkey kicks:
Start on all-fours. Brace your core and lift one leg up keeping the knee bent and the sole of the foot flat towards the ceiling. Bring it back down to the start position and do desired number of reps before changing sides **(easier option: reduce the range of leg movement).**

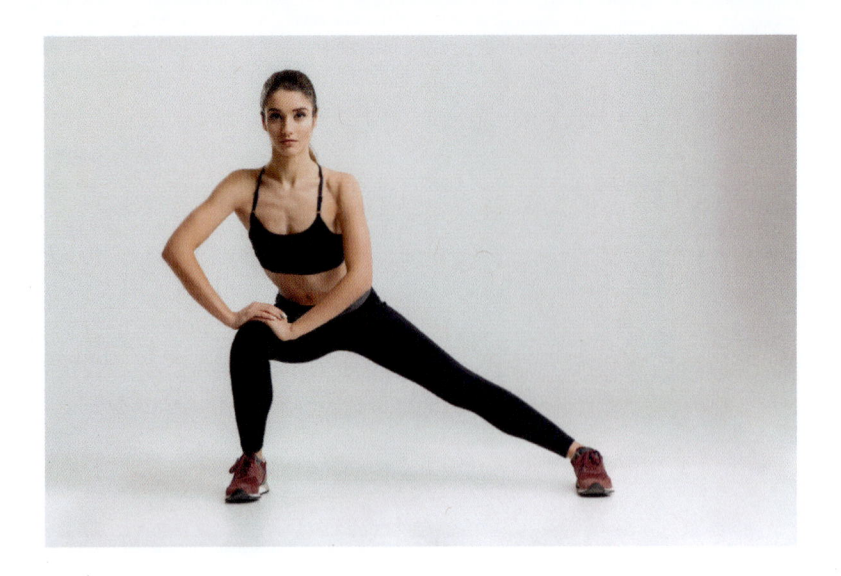

Static Side lunges:
Stand tall and take a big step to the side until the knee of that leg is bent to around 90 degrees whilst keeping your trailing leg straight. Push back up to the start position and repeat on the other side **(easier option: take leading knee to 45 degrees).**

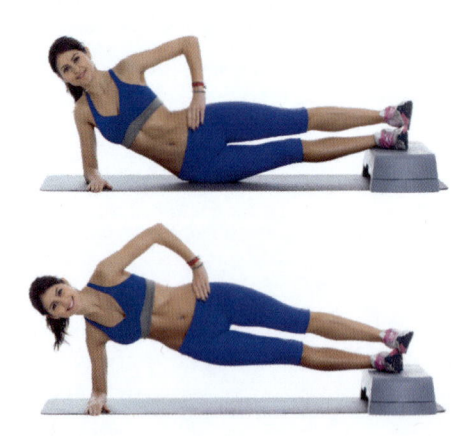

Side plank hip dip:
Assume a side-lying position with your forearm resting on the floor (elevate your legs to make it harder). Push up from the elbow so your hips are raised and form a straight line from your shoulders through your ankles. Dip the hips as near to the floor as you can and return to the top **(easier option: bend your knees and/or keep them on the floor).**

Flexibility (or limberness) relates to the range of movement in a joint or joints, and in the length of the muscle that crosses those joints.

When you're a child, flexibility comes easily. When you're an adult you have to work to maintain and improve it. Over the age of 50 and the goal posts change altogether because the body goes through natural deterioration that leads to compromised movement. The decline includes: loss of muscle mass, loss of bone density, decrease in tendons' water content, decrease in elasticity of ligaments and a thinning of cartilage between joints. The knock-on effect of these things includes stiffness, pain, weakness and reduced functionality.

If you're over 50 you probably know what I mean. You get out of bed in the morning and it's a challenge to walk to the bathroom without something hurting. As you get older it gets worse and if you don't do something about it, you'll reach the point where you can't bend down to pick something up or get out of your chair. The antidote to a lack of flexibility/stiffness is stretching — regularly.

29

DO STRETCHES FOR IMPROVED FLEXIBILITY, INCLUDING THE FOLLOWING

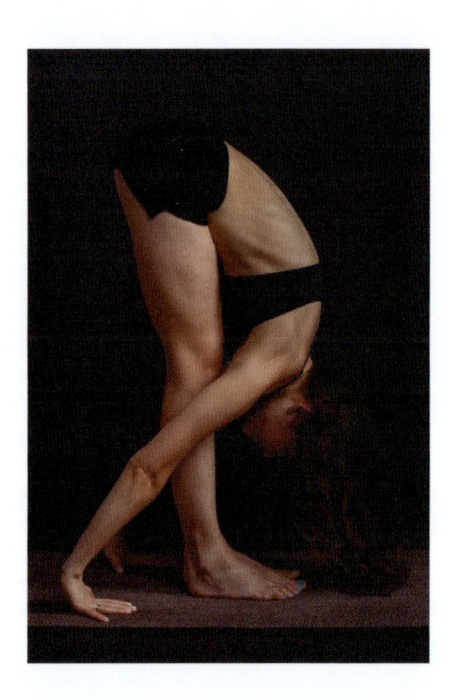

Forward stretch:
Stand tall, bend from the waist bringing your chest towards your thighs. Keep your legs straight. Reach for the floor with straight arms. It doesn't matter if you can't get all the way down. At the bottom, take two deep breaths before coming slowly back up. This stretches the lower back and the hamstrings.

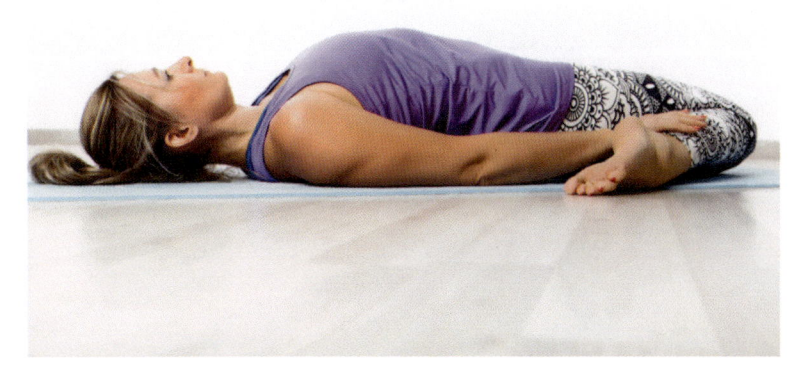

Side knee tilts/rolls:
Lie on your back with your knees raised to a 90-degree angle. Slowly tilt them over to one side until they reach the floor, or as near as you can get. Keep your knees and feet together and ensure your shoulders stay on the floor. Hold for at least ten-seconds. This stretches the hips, lower back and waist.

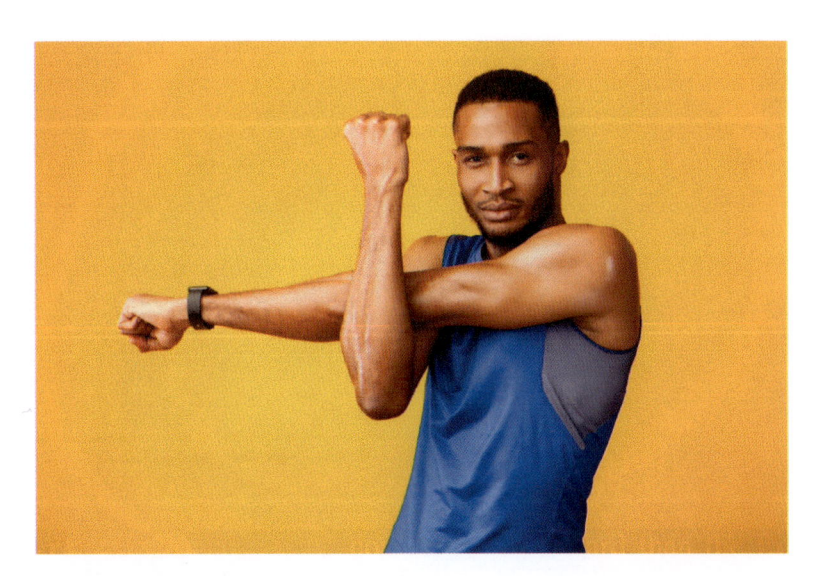

Standing shoulder stretch:
Take one arm across your body and cradle the elbow with your other hand. Keep the shoulder below the ear and look over the shoulder that you're stretching for tension release in the neck.

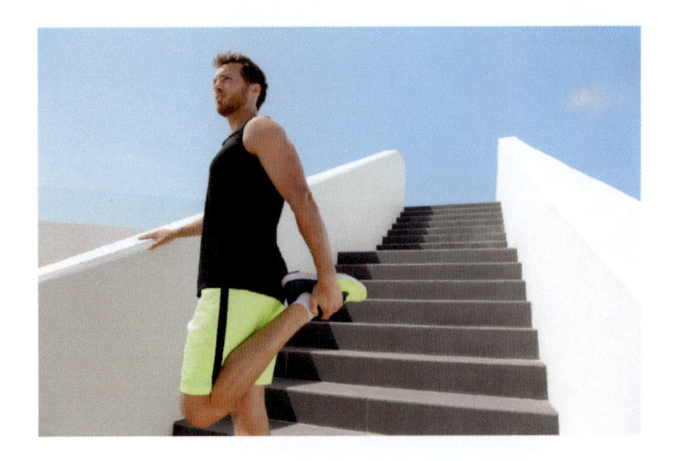

Standing Quad stretch:
Stand tall with your feet close together. Lift one knee backwards and grip the front of that foot with the free hand.
Hold for at least 20 seconds ensuring your knees are together, your hips are pushed forward, and your shoulders are back. Lower gently, repeat on the other side.

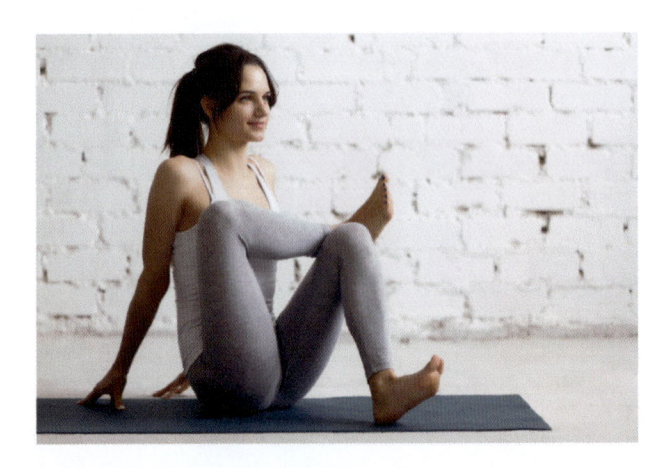

Glute stretch:
Sit on a chair, or the floor. Cross one leg over the other and then use your hand to pull up the foot of the crossed leg to rest on the opposite thigh. Hold for at least 20 seconds before lowering and changing sides. If you have good balance, this can also be done in a standing position: adopt the same pose and crouch down, bending the supporting knee as you go.

If you've done the maths, you'll know that if you complete each of the suggested exercises in each of the categories, you will end up doing 30 exercises. The stretches, however, are best done at the end as part of a cool down.

It is, of course, up to you how you divide them up or if you want to add exercises of your own, but either way you may be wondering how long to do each of them for and how much rest to take between them.

There's no right or wrong answer to this question and it very much depends on personal factors such as your fitness level or the amount of time you have to do a workout. But almost all the recent studies that have looked at varying systems of exercise in terms of their efficiency have concluded that High Intensity Interval Training (HIIT) works best in terms of results for most people. I agree.

30

INCLUDE HITT TRAINING IN YOUR EXERCISE PLAN

I know the words that make up the acronym HIIT (High Intensity Interval Training) are scary, and I suspect you might be thinking: I'm over 50 and unfit, HIIT's not for me. WRONG! HIIT is for almost any one of any age and fitness. That is because you can customise the times of work and rest to suit your abilities.

Essentially what HIIT means is alternating short periods of hard work with specific rest times in-between. The rest times can be longer, shorter or the same as the work times. **What's matters is how *hard* you work, not how *long* you work.**

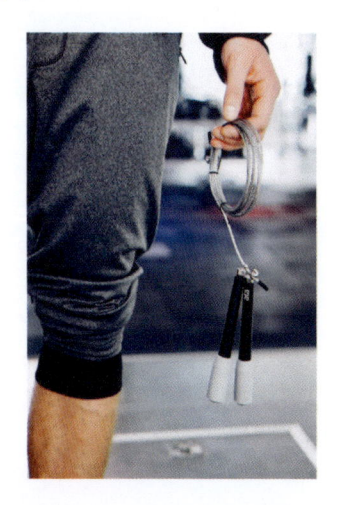

When you spend a long time doing some form of exercise — for e.g. running at a constant pace around your local park — it does help your general fitness, but it's more geared towards improving your stamina and endurance. It's a different type of training known as Low Intensity Steady State (LISS). There is certainly a place for it alongside (or instead) of HIIT training, but for now we're going to focus on HIIT.

Here are some suggested work-rest combinations:

- If you're new to exercise and unfit, you may want to start doing each exercise for 15-20 seconds with 35-40 seconds rest before the next.
- If you have a rudimentary level of fitness you could try 30 seconds per exercise with 40 rest.
- As you improve you might choose to extend the exercise to 40 seconds with 30 seconds of rest.
- After that, you could try 45 seconds with 25 seconds' rest.
- And, when you're really fit, you can experiment with less rest time than work time.

The combinations are numerous, so play around with them to find what's appropriate for you.

The other thing to consider is whether you want to do a particular exercise once or more than once (known as a set)

So, for example, if one day you wanted to concentrate on your abs and core, you could choose to do each exercise multiple times – say five times each. Even then you have a choice, you could do each of your five exercises once then repeat the pattern five times or do each exercise five times before moving onto the next.

The great thing about HIIT is that you don't have to spend ages doing it. Many HIIT workouts last 20 minutes — and that's enough IF you've been working at an intensity that's high enough. What this means is that you go all-out during the work time, but never fully recover before embarking on the next exercise. By the end of the session you should be really tired, and your heart rate should be really high.

The other advantage of HIIT compared to many other types of exercise is that you get an after-burn effect called EPOC (excess post exercise oxygen consumption). What this means is that your heart rate remains elevated after you've stopped training so that you continue to burn calories and fat.

HIIT is often associated with cardio rather than other types of exercise but it can also be applied to any sort of training in which repetition (reps) of exercise is involved.

Play around with formulas to find what works for you. For example, you may choose to do HIIT for your cardio and resistance exercises and a specific number of reps for other categories such as hips-thighs-glutes. Either way, make sure you monitor how much work and how much rest you're doing so that the workout has a proper structure.

Before you do any exercise, you need to prepare the body for it, and afterwards, it needs to relax.

31

ALWAYS WARM UP AND COOL DOWN

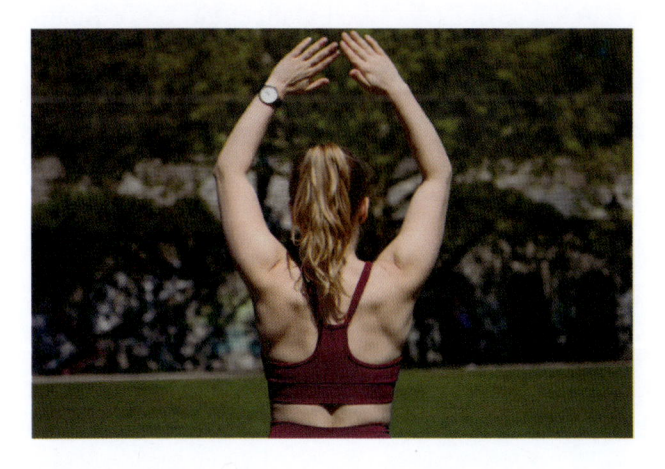

It never ceases to amaze me how many people go straight into hardcore exercise the moment they step into a gym/workout space - even seasoned exercisers who should know better.
Yes, I know, warming-up is a bit of a bind, it adds time to a workout you want to do quickly because you're short of time, but it's IMPORTANT and you should consider it PART of your workout.

In essence, a warm up prepares the body for the workload coming its way while decreasing the chance of injury. Specifically, it:

- **Increases body temperature** which prompts the heart to pump more blood more rapidly around the body to the places where it's going to be needed.

- **Improves joint safety** by working gently on their range of motion to make them more flexible. Immobile joints make it hard to move properly and stiff joints are vulnerable to injury.
- **Speeds up the flow of blood to tissues** which results in greater muscle flexibility. The more elastic a muscle, the less chance it has of being strained or torn.
- **Triggers hormonal changes** that boost metabolism. What this means is that the body makes available it's carbohydrate and fat sources for energy. This also affects the production of excess lactic acid which can accumulate in the blood and makes exercise feel a lot harder than it should because your muscles feel like they're 'burning.' (this is why sometimes for the first few minutes of a workout, the exertion feels unmanageable).
- **Prepares you mentally** and boosts the nervous system which helps with skills like balance and co-ordination.

A warm up should mimic the type of the workout you are about to do, but there should always be exercises to increase your heart rate and stretch and mobilise your muscles. So if, for example, you are planning to do a lower body weights workout, you might want to do various squats and lunges without weights. Then, you could choose four or five gentle cardio exercises – such as jogging on the spot – before finishing with some dynamic stretching (stretching as you move) and some joint mobilisation work, e.g. shoulder rotations.

For an average length workout, a warm up should last at least five minutes. When it's finished take a short rest and some water before you start properly.

A **cool down** is as important as a warm up. It enables the body to safely return to its pre-workout state. If you stop abruptly the blood can pool in your muscles (notably the legs) and make you feel sick or faint.

Specifically, it decreases the heart rate, brings down blood pressure, removes waste products such as lactic acid and can prevent stiffness or soreness over the next 48 hours.

Stretching is the most effective way to cool down because it addresses the above issues. Concentrate on stretching the muscles you have been working the most. So, if you only did an upper body workout, focus on muscles above the waist including the shoulders, biceps, triceps and neck.

Another reason for stretching is that the repetitive action of many forms of exercise – for e.g. running – can create a muscular imbalance if stretching is not included. Over time this can cause pain and posture problems – particularly in the lower back.

And breathe…the other important aspect of a cool down is that it allows you and your muscles to relax. Exhale as you ease into a stretch and inhale on the way back. Stretch to the point of tension, not pain.

It's ok for the cool down to be slightly shorter than the warm up, but I suggest not less than five minutes.

Exercise takes many forms and HIIT is just one. It does, however, reflect sections of the Government's physical activity guidelines which state that an **adult between the ages of 19 and 64 should do at least 150 minutes of moderate intensity activity a week or 75 minutes of vigorous intensity activity a week.**

The other main recommendation is that all adults should do strengthening exercise that works all the major muscle groups (legs, hips, back, abdomen, chest, shoulders and arms) on at least two days a week.

The only separate things the Government advocates for people over the age of 65 is that they incorporate balance and flexibility exercise into their strength work.

My suggested plan is a little more ambitious, but it needs to be, if you're going to control your weight AND become really fit and healthy.

If you do what I recommend three to four times a week for around 30-45 minutes per session (including the warm up and cool down) you should start seeing results in weeks rather than months. Combined with a healthy, calorie conscious diet, it's likely be sooner.

The key thing about exercise is this: it's a journey without a destination. The aim is not to arrive at a particular point which signifies the end. The aim is to carry on doing it for as long as you're physically able.

If you stop, so too will the benefits — not immediately, but it won't take long. Also, the gains you made will disappear a lot quicker than they took to acquire and when/if your re-start, it will feel like an uphill struggle to get back to where you were.

One way to make exercise sustainable is to keep it interesting. So:

32

INCLUDE EXERCISE VARIETY IN YOUR PLAN

If you do the same thing every day/week/month, you'll get bored and eventually give up. This applies to many aspects of life including exercise. Obviously, there's some things you can't give up for practical reasons e.g. your job, but it's very easy to give up exercise because most people don't consider it essential and, let's face it, what's more appealing — a night in front of the TV with a pizza, or a gruelling workout at the gym!?

So, find different types of exercise that you enjoy and incorporate them into your plan.

If you're looking at the Government guidelines and wondering what counts as moderate intensity activity, then consider: brisk walking/gentle jogging, water aerobics, bike riding, dancing, golf, yoga, pushing a lawn mower and housework.

And the following things count as vigorous activity: running fast, swimming, riding a bike uphill, group exercise classes like 'aerobics', rope skipping and sports like football, table tennis or squash.

Also be aware that although it's obviously better to do something than nothing, certain types of activity — such as regular pace walking — can really only be counted as 'movement' or low-level activity.

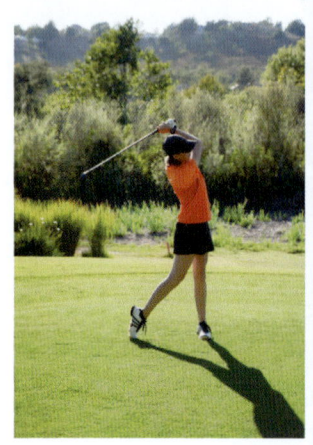

CASE STUDY 2
David, 70

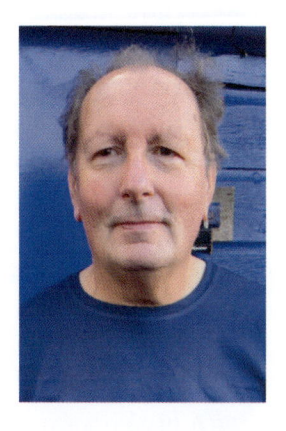

David had always been active and enjoyed walking and cycling as well as sports including tennis, which he played regularly. As he got older, however, he realised he was running out of puff as he ran round the tennis court and he began to worry other aspects of his health and fitness were deteriorating. Keen not to let the trend continue, he decided to join a gym…only when he got there, he wasn't sure what to do, so he started attending Pilates classes which opened his eyes to the wonders and benefits of structured exercise.

When I started training David at the age of 67, he was a little overweight and had slightly high blood pressure. He informed me was taking statins to stabilise his cholesterol levels healthy and that his goals included increasing general fitness and building muscle, particularly in his upper body. When he started working out, he realised that other things he had previously taken for granted, or not considered, were an issue.

David, a book binder, said: "I thought I was fairly fit for my age because I could play tennis up to five times a week and I was rarely ill. But I soon came to realise that fitness covers a broad spectrum of things, many of which I hadn't even thought about.

> "I thought being stiff, inflexible and unbalanced were just symptoms of getting older, something I had to put up with. But over time and with practice I came to understand that they can be improved and I'm so happy they have been. It makes everyday tasks a lot easier."

David says after just a few sessions in the gym he felt changes taking place.

> "I was in my late 60s and had never run on a treadmill before, I thought that sort of thing was for someone in their 20's. I was a little nervous at first but soon got the hang of it and within a few months was running continuously at varying speeds for over 10 minutes. Also, lifting weights was a revelation. I didn't know there was so many different exercises for so many different parts of the body. After a while I was lifting heavier and for longer and I could feel and see improvements in muscle strength."

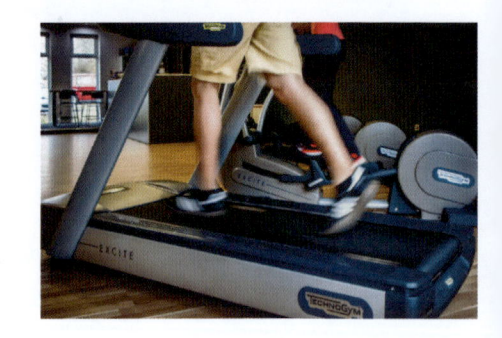

David, who now trains in the gym once or twice a week (as well as playing tennis up to five times a week) added:

> "At first I was completely exhausted after workouts, but it didn't take long for my energy levels to improve — both in and out of the gym. It got me thinking how I'd taken my health and fitness for granted and how I would never do so again.
> I now look at some of my friends who aren't fit or healthy — either because of an inactive lifestyle or illness — and feel grateful that I'm not in that position. As you get older, life is certainly harder without your health. Workouts now fly by and the variety of things I do means my whole body is being kept in shape — for e.g. my core and abs are stronger which gives my stomach a better shape. The sense of achievement after a hard workout should be acknowledged too. If I start the session with any negativity, by the end it's been pushed out."

David concludes:

> "You may not be able to turn back time, but I believe you can hold back physical and mental decline. I also know I'll still be able to walk up the stairs when I'm 90 which is a relief!"

33

TO WALK OR NOT TO WALK? AND DO YOU REALLY NEED TO DO 10,000 STEPS A DAY?

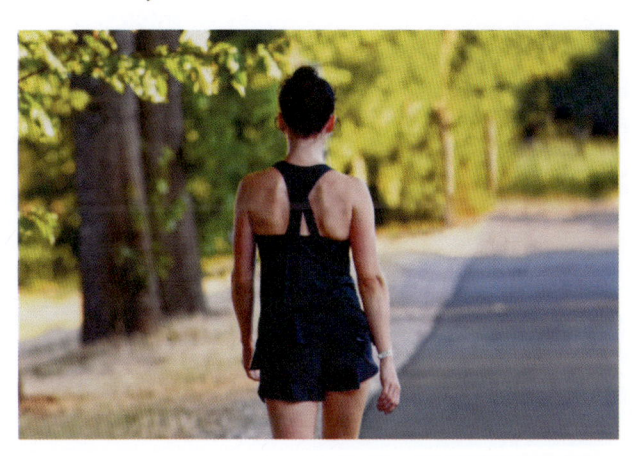

If you're *not* doing any other exercise walking is important because 10,000 daily steps roughly equates to one of the Government's recommended activity targets of 2.5 hours of moderate intensity exercise a week.

But if you are doing regular exercise, it may not be an issue because you'll almost certainly be getting your quota in a different way.

Ten thousand steps roughly equates to five miles. The average British person walks between 3,000 and 4,000 steps a day, so there will be a deficit for most people.

If you have a busy life, it's not going to be easy to find the time to do it and, if you're not into walking, you may not be motivated to do it. If this is the case, I believe you'd be far better off doing the sort of exercise I recommend in this book.

Clearly, it's a personal choice and you could decide, for example, to do 10,000 steps on the days you're not doing other types of exercise.

Fortunately, steps don't only refer to putting one foot in front of the other in the form of conventional walking. Other activities count too.

Here's a quick guide to everyday things that contribute towards your step quota. The numbers refer to steps per minute:

- Washing the car: 75
- Vacuuming: 90
- Slow cycling: 93
- Playing golf: 100
- Fast dancing: 150
- Heavy gardening: 155

To ensure accuracy it's best to use a pedometer, a fitness tracker or there's plenty of apps available via your smartphone. The NHS has one, it's called Active 10.

A final word about walking: it is, of course, good for you and it's free and easy to do. But if walking is your only form of exercise and you do it periodically at a leisurely pace for short distances it probably won't have a great effect on your health and fitness and you're unlikely to lose weight.

To use it as a more effective exercise tool, you need to walk regularly, briskly and for longer distances so that you feel slightly out of breath whilst doing it. This indicates you're getting a cardio benefit and burning calories.

Walking briskly for 30 minutes could burn 150-200 calories. If you do that every day, that's a total of approximately 1,250 calories a week. Depending on your diet, you could well be creating a calorie deficit which would, over time, lead to weight loss. To make it more challenging, why not carry some light dumbbells and do some upper body exercises as you go?

34

GO JOGGING OR RUNNING, BUT LISTEN TO YOUR BODY

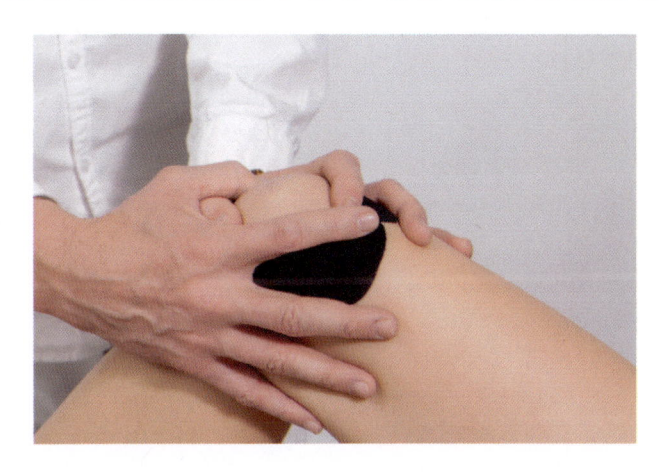

When you're next in the park on a Saturday morning, take a look around at the people running and you will notice that lots of them are wearing knee or other types of supports.

Not the young runners, they don't need to, their joints aren't wearing out yet, but those over the age of about 40 – many of whom have been pounding the streets for years – cannot run without one (or two in some cases) because it's so painful. It's a common sight and if this is you, I urge you to either stop or cut back on your running and find an alternate form of exercise. If you don't, you may well end up immobile and on a very long waiting list for a knee replacement. Ditto for other joints antagonised by running such as your hip.

Running can be a two-edged sword; it's a great form of cardio exercise, it's free, it's simple and it gets you outdoors when you otherwise might not bother. Running on a treadmill works in much the same way.

Running's good for strengthening your legs, butt and core and it's beneficial for your bones because the weight bearing aspect of the movement causes them to become stronger and denser. However, the flip side of this is that running is a high impact repetitive movement and if you do it regularly (or too much), you can cause injuries such as shin splints, stress fractures, strains and sprains. This occurs more as you get older and is particularly common if you have joint or muscle vulnerabilities.

On top of that, as you age, the wear and tear on your joints and muscles can lead to localised pain and soreness (without having a specific injury). This not only takes the joy out of running, but it also makes it inefficient as other areas of your body compensate for the discomfort, potentially causing a separate set of problems connected with muscle imbalance.

If you're new to running and want a great way to build up your ability, then look no further than a plan called **Couch to 5k** which has become known around the world. There are various versions of it, but essentially, it's a nine week scheme aimed at getting couch potatoes off their butts and running 5k (3.1 miles) within just over two months. The early weeks combine walking, jogging and running but by the end, it's just running. It's incredibly popular because it works, and it doesn't feel too arduous. I know many people who have used it successfully, some of whom now do half marathons. The NHS does it as a podcast and an app which you can access via their **NHS Choices website.**

If you want your fitness to keep improving (why wouldn't you?) It's crucial that you don't keep doing the same thing over and over again. After a while, your body will get used to it and no longer makes the adaptations required to reap the benefits. So:

35

MAKE SURE PROGRESSIVE OVERLOAD IS PART OF YOUR PLAN

Progressive overload is a fancy way of saying do things regularly to make your workout harder. More specifically, it refers to gradually overloading the body with either intensity, volume, frequency or time in order to improve.

If, for example, at the beginning of your exercise regime you decide to do two sets of 10 bicep curls with 3 kg dumbbells because that challenges you, after 12 months you would almost certainly find it quite easy. That's because your body has adapted to make your biceps stronger. If you then do nothing, your biceps will not change (because they don't have to in order to perform the exercise) If, however, you increase the weight to 4 kg and do three sets of 12 reps, it will feel challenging again and your body will have to adjust to the new demands and therefore get stronger.

Progressive overload is often associated with strength training — whereby you gradually increase the weight of what you're lifting over time.

But the term can — and should be — applied to any form of exercise because you can always make it more testing by increasing one or more aspects of it.

Besides the physical effects, your brain also gets a boost from progressive overload. Doing something that's become easy numbs and distracts the mind. In order to find the strength to do something more challenging, your brain must focus.

36

IMPROVE YOUR POSTURE

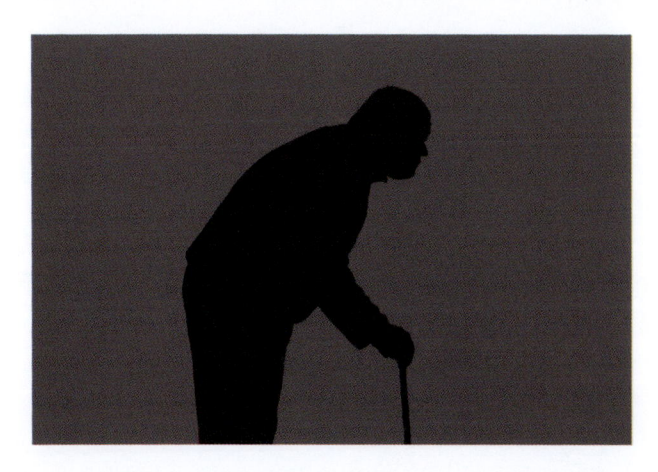

It's a sad sight, a little old lady/man hunched over and struggling to walk. You wonder how she/he got to that stage and hope it doesn't happen to you.

The good news is that it doesn't have to, and if you work on your posture, it won't — unless you have a degenerative spine condition, osteoporosis or similar. While it is a normal part of ageing to become slightly less erect (due to diminishing bone density and vertebrae disc erosion altering gravitational forces) it is compounded by a more modern phenomenon — sitting hunched over a computer and/or phone all day. Bad posture makes for more bad posture. This is because your muscles and ligaments are put under so much strain, they're unable to work as nature intended and they become mis-aligned. This can then affect your vital organs which are effectively 'pushed' out of their proper position as well as your immune and digestive system. Long term, it can compromise efficient breathing. There are some simple things you can do to improve your posture, and I recommend everyone over the age of 50 does them.

Stand up straight:
In good, standing posture, your head, shoulders, hips and ankles are aligned. Your eyes are facing forward, your chin is up, and your shoulders are back and slightly down, lined up with your ears. Your weight is evenly distributed from the back to the front of your feet and your core is tight (think sucking in your belly button towards your spine)

Sit up straight:
Particularly at your computer and have your screen at an appropriate distance – close enough that you don't have to tilt forward to read and far enough away to lessen the glare. Take a break at least every 30 minutes. Have a walk round and stretch your legs and back.

Try not to cross your legs for long periods:
This makes your hips uneven and leads to muscular tension in the back up to the neck. It can also affect your pelvis and, ultimately, the way you walk.

Exercise regularly:
Almost all exercise helps your posture because you strengthen muscles that support your spine. Focus on your core and glutes, and work on your balance and range of movement. Excellent ways to do this include yoga and Pilates.

37

PUSH YOURSELF, BUT DON'T BURNOUT

If a little exercise is good for you, more must be better, right? And, in general, this is true.

But there is a tipping point beyond which the more exercise your do, the more harm it can do. It's called overtraining and it's very real.

By all means push yourself to your limits during the workout. In fact you should. The maxim 'no pain, no gain' is spot on where intensity and endurance within a workout is concerned, but you absolutely must get enough rest between sessions for your body to recover enough to perform at an equally intense - or higher - level next time. There is no magic formula for how much exercise is too much. Levels will vary from person to person based on existing health and fitness, age, medical conditions or injuries, stress levels, sleep and diet, amongst other things.

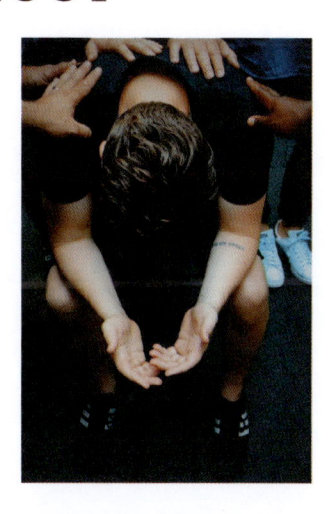

But if you experience more than one of the following symptoms you should ask yourself if you're overdoing it:

- Extreme fatigue or unexplained weakness
- A decrease in your exercise performance
- Chronic muscle soreness, pain or strain that doesn't go away
- Reduced appetite and weight loss
- Irritability and anxiety
- Sleep problems
- Weight gain (overtraining messes up your hormones. The body produces too much of the stress hormone cortisol which prompts the body to hold onto calories and fat)
- Lack of motivation. Working out becomes a massive chore you no longer enjoy

Instinct and self-awareness should also tell you if you're overtraining, so listen to your body and mind. If you're burned out, the best thing to do is stop for a while. I suggest at least two weeks. Your body needs this amount of time to recover and re-set. Alternatively, find a gentler more holistic form of exercise, such as yoga, for a while.

There's seven days in a week. No one should be training every day of the week — not even elite athletes. If you're new to exercise, I recommend at least one day's rest between each session. If you're a seasoned exerciser, there's nothing to stop you training on consecutive days, but I advise no more than five out of seven days a week.

38

KNOW THAT EXERCISE SHORTCUTS DO NOT EXIST AND BEWARE OF FADS/GADGETS

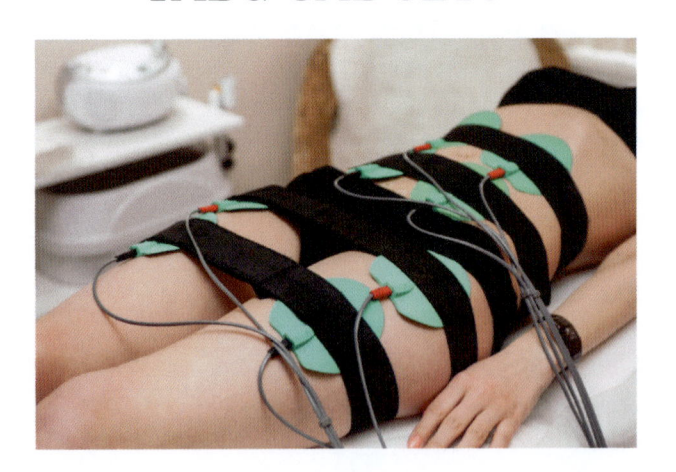

If you're a woman over 50, you may recall what was dubbed a 'miracle' form of exercise back in the 80's.

I won't state the brand name, but the 'miracle' involved placing sticky pads over various parts of your body and flicking a switch that sent electrical impulses into your muscles to strengthen and tone them.

I remember it well because I bought one, hoping it would mean I didn't have to exercise (I hadn't caught the exercise bug back then). I used to sit in front of the TV with my feet up for hours, just waiting for the magic to work.

Here's what happened…NOTHING and it was painful. I knew a few women who had the same experience, and they all gave up on it.

News alert: the technology has recently made a comeback. It's been updated and given a makeover whereby you can now wear it in belt or 'body suit' form and it's known generically as EMS – Electrical Muscle Stimulation.

Different companies have different products, but they all claim much the same thing – that clinical studies show that if you use it as prescribed, you'll see results within around a month. By results, they mean inch loss, muscle definition or dropping a dress size.

I'm sure it does work for some people, but there's certain biological facts that go hand in hand with real exercise that EMS simply can't replicate and that goes for the numerous other exercise-substitute gadgets out there.

A selection that spring to mind that I would include in this category are vibrating power plates, power-balance hologram bracelets, toning training shoes, weighted knives and forks, and sauna -suits.

Remember the old adage, if something sounds too good to be true, it probably is.

FOOT NOTE: there's no reason why you can't incorporate some of these things into a fitness regime on a complementary basis. They can also be helpful to people with limited mobility.

39

CONSIDER USING LESS WELL-KNOWN KIT IN YOUR WORKOUTS

Stability ball:
Also known as a Swiss or mobility ball, this is particularly useful for abs, core, glutes, balance and stability work.

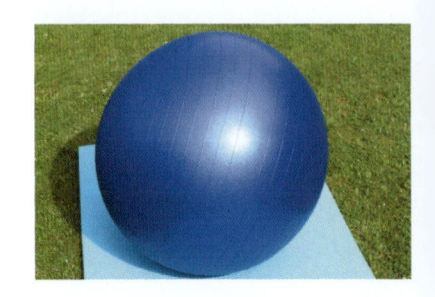

Step:
Use for cardio/conditioning work. Start by stepping up and down and progress to more ambitious things like jumps and press ups.

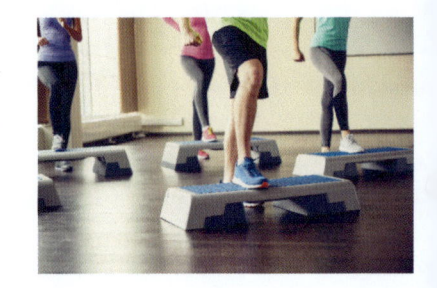

Medicine Ball:
Never try to kick a medicine ball, you'll break your foot! For those of you who don't know, it's a weighted ball (there are varying degrees of heaviness) which can be used in similar ways to dumbbells.

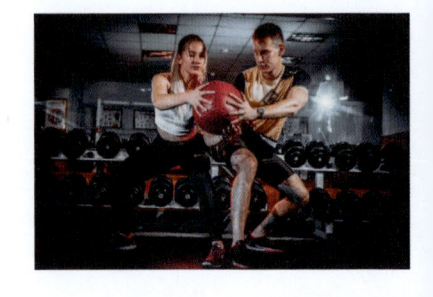

Kettlebell:
Kettlebell swings are considered one of the best full body exercises you can do. They are excellent for conditioning your core and improving your flexibility and movement patterns.

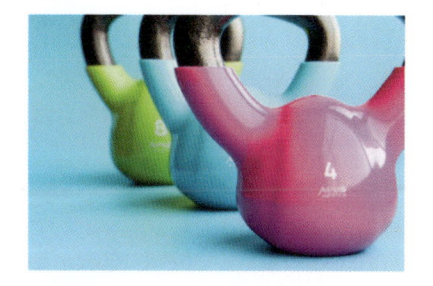

VIPR: (an acronym which stands for Vitality, Performance, Re-conditioning) This bit of kit bridges the gap between movement and strength training with the additional benefit of improving agility. Often used in exercises that work the shoulders, back and core.

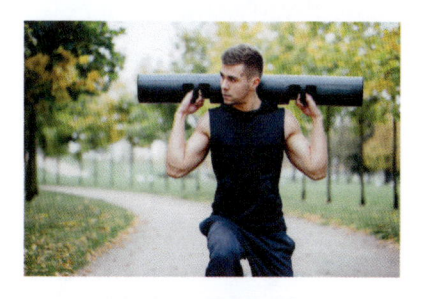

Skipping Rope:
There's a reason why boxers are super-fit…they do a lot of skipping. It's perfect for raising your heart rate, not to mention strengthening your legs.

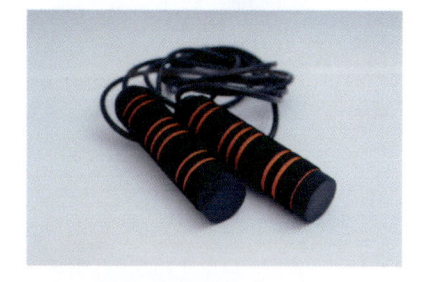

Barbell:
An ideal way to add resistance to squats, lunges and deadlifts, it's also hugely beneficial for upper body work such as upright rows.

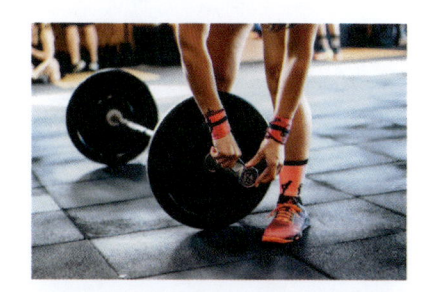

Plyobox:
Plyo is short for plyometrics — which essentially means explosive movement, particularly jumping. You don't have to jump though, you can start by stepping up and down. Plastic rather than wood boxes are best, in my opinion.

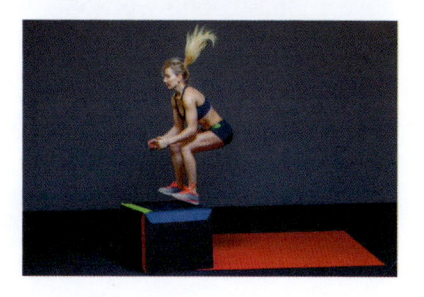

Resistance Band:
First considered a bit of a craze, now a must-have for anyone trying to boost their booty. Bands can be used in many different ways, but they work best placed round the mid thighs when training the butt with squats. The fabric type are far better than the rubber ones.

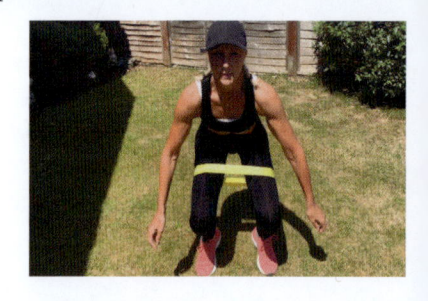

Battle Ropes:
Exercise is a series of battles, mainly with yourself, and this bit off kit goes a long way towards winning the war. Battle ropes work your entire body. They help build strength and enable you to torch calories and fat in a fun and unusual way.

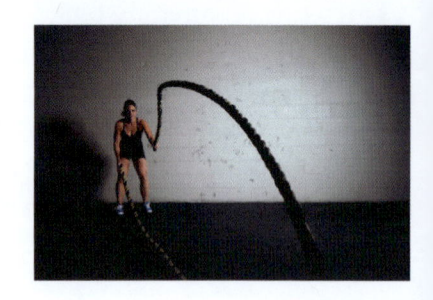

40
GET A PERSONAL TRAINER

I would say that, wouldn't I!?

But, in all honesty, I wouldn't say it unless I thought it was a bona fide point. There are a number of indisputable advantages of having one-to-one workouts with an accredited professional. The first and perhaps most important is that a PT can devise a bespoke programme tailored to your needs and abilities that is both safe and efficient.

I see people in the gym all the time who clearly don't know what they're doing.

They either have terrible technique which could lead to injury or they don't know how to use a particular piece of equipment. There are

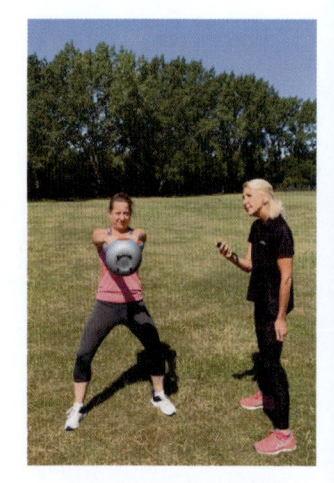

Me. training a client

others who come to the gym day after day, year after year, and do exactly the same thing in exactly the same order. Not only must that be mind numbingly boring, but the law of diminishing returns means they won't be getting as much benefit as they think they are.

The next big advantage of having a PT is that she/he will motivate you. If you've booked and paid for a session, you're going to show up for it – that's the first hurdle crossed. Then, during the session, your PT will use motivational techniques designed to make you push yourself harder than you would if you were alone.

What this inevitably leads to are quicker results. Some PTs shout, some PTS coerce and some PTs have a softly, softly touch. Whatever their characteristics you can be sure a good PT will have acquired a sense of who you are and how best you need to be trained.

If you are recovering from an injury or other condition, a PT can make a huge difference to your rehabilitation. Not only can they incorporate exercises that help heal the issue, but they can ensure you don't suffer further injury.

I once trained a lady well over the age of 50 who broke her leg badly. When I first met her she was on crutches and could barely walk. We started with chair exercises just using her bodyweight and soon progressed to exercises on the chair using dumbbells. A few weeks into the programme she was on her feet with one crutch, a few weeks later, no crutch at all and in less than a year I had her running and jumping about. She was so pleased with her progress, she persuaded her husband to join in and I trained them both. I was heartened to see her transformation, not to mention her husband's.

A PT plays a part in your own accountability. A good PT will have taken baseline health and fitness statistics (of the sort mentioned earlier in the book) when you started, and will review your progress regularly. The fact you know the appraisals are upcoming, means you're more likely to keep yourself on track.

A PT can make exercise interesting and fun. I go out of my way to make all my clients' session unlike the previous one: different exercises, different formats different reps, different intervals and different pieces of equipment. This keeps them on their toes and they normally react with energy and enthusiasm. Often, I include 'fun' challenges like how long they can hold a low squat with a dumbbell.

Believe it or not, your PT can become your friend. I'm not talking about someone you can go on holiday with, I'm talking about another human being who knows and gets you. Someone who has your best interests at heart and someone you can trust. Feeling supported can help with your confidence and self esteem.

A PT should also inspire and mentor you. I don't know any fat, unfit personal trainers and I can tell you from my own experience, that we train hard in order to maintain a body, mind and lifestyle others want to emulate.

In conclusion, if you can afford a personal trainer, do get one. But make sure it's the right one for you. There are lots of good ones out there and lots of bad ones.

Be aware the good ones might not be good for *you*. Personal training is just that – personal. It's about personality and building rapport to build results. Do your research (e.g. check qualifications) and before you hand over a big wad of money, do an introductory session, after which you can decide whether you're a good fit for each other.

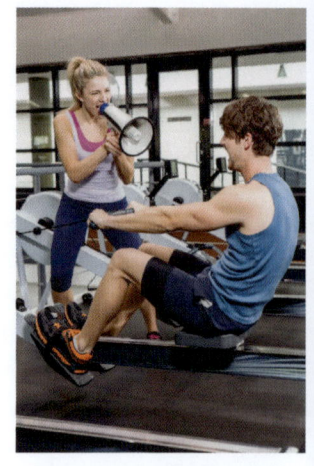

Make sure the PT is right for you

CASE STUDY 3
Anne, 65

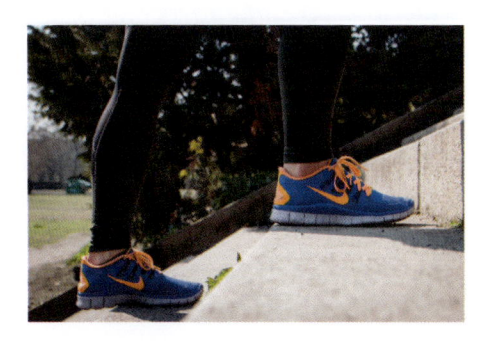

As a personal trainer for many years, I've worked with hundreds of people from all walks of life. When they start an exercise programme, they tend to fall in one of four categories:

1. Those with bags of enthusiasm who remain that way
2. Those who are super-keen but drop out when the novelty wears off
3. Those who start reluctantly but turn into exercise converts
4. Those who start half-heartedly and never really change

And then there's Anne…in a category all of her own!

I have never known anyone so averse to the idea of exercise and never have I encountered a client who complains as much as she does while doing it. During sessions she clock watches, employs time wasting strategies she thinks I'm not aware of and tries to cheat on the hard exercises in a bid to make them easier.

But you know what, this has been going on for four years and despite her quirks, she actually ends up working really hard and is committed to the process. Unlike most other clients, she's never cancelled any of her twice weekly sessions and she now exercises on her own at home. And the best part for both of us is – she's made amazing gains in her health and fitness.

This is her story:

"I've always hated exercise and loved food. In my youth this wasn't a problem. I was very slim, played squash and

badminton to club standard and never had to worry about my weight or fitness. Over the years my work-life balance shifted until I was fully occupied with long working hours which meant I had very little time to exercise. By the time I retired I had discovered the pleasure of playing golf, but I was also about a stone heavier than I wanted to be and struggling with a painful knee condition which eventually required surgery.

On top of this I had many personal stresses and heavy family commitments which meant life had most definitely got in the way of living well. All I could do was cope with situations rather than contemplate changing them. After a while, however, my weight had got to its 'go no further limit', so I did what all women did, I went on a diet – more than one actually – and I did shed some weight. But every time I stopped, I re-gained and felt I was back to square one. It soon dawned on me with dreaded realisation that I needed to exercise."

Former deputy head teacher Anne joined a gym and started doing group exercise classes. She says:

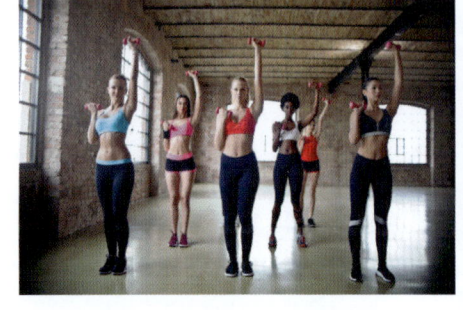

"I hated them with a passion, I couldn't bear being in a room full of young gym bunnies when quite obviously I wasn't one. So, I decided to adopt a different strategy and look for a personal trainer. Fortunately I struck lucky finding Aylia. She was interested in a holistic approach to overall health and fitness and encouraged me to understand that diet, exercise and the mind are inextricably linked in terms of weight loss. She described this concept as Tri-Hybrid-Health©.

Anne couldn't bear gym bunnies

Until this point, I was always tackling one or the other in isolation. Being trained by a professional was not a 'road to Damascus' experience. My attitude to exercise itself didn't really change, but other things did. It was pointed out to me that a PT could lead me to fitness, but the results were down to me, so I decided to commit to the process. It helped to have someone standing over me issuing instructions. I didn't always like it, but I realised it was a case of being cruel to be kind!"

Anne lost more than half a stone in weight by not 'going on a diet' but by modifying her diet.

Her method meant she increased her good-carb and protein intake and reduced her fat consumption. She served up smaller portion sizes and snacked less. She reduced her alcohol consumption but still allowed herself a couple of glasses of wine a week, and if she had a craving for chocolate, she indulged it by having a square or two rather than the bar she would have opted for before.

Soon her fitness hugely improved. During our first ever training session, she had to keep sitting down and, at one point, thought she was going to pass out. Now, she can keep up a high intensity exercise for more than a minute without a problem (something many of my much younger clients can't).

Anne's posture is also better. When I met her, she walked with her head down and her shoulders hunched over. Thanks to the natural course of exercise, she now stands a little taller (and prouder).

Interestingly, a positive turning point for Anne came after an elongated period of inactivity due to the COVID-19 pandemic. On her return to exercise she decided to change her sessions from one hour to 45 minutes and the training was conducted via Zoom rather than in the gym.

She concludes:

> *"I'll never be a gym bunny who loves exercise, but I've gone from telling myself that 'I hate this,' to 'I can do this,' and that's a massive step. I've been spurred on by doing it from my home where I feel comfortable. The way things are going, I'll be 'fit, not fat, after 50' for many years to come!"*

PART THREE

THE MIND AND MENTAL HEALTH

The final section looks at health and fitness from a psychological perspective. Exercise, nutrition and brain health are inextricably linked; one influences the other in either a positive or negative way. A healthy brain leads to a healthy life, just as much as a healthy body does…and vice versa. So which should be the priority?

The answer is – none of them. You should look after them all with equal resolve. Back in the day, being 'well' simply meant the 'absence of disease.' Thankfully we're more enlightened in the 21st Century and although the term 'wellness' has become so broad that it can lack definition, I suspect most people now agree that it unequivocally involves mental health.

41

EXERCISE TO IMPROVE YOUR MENTAL HEALTH

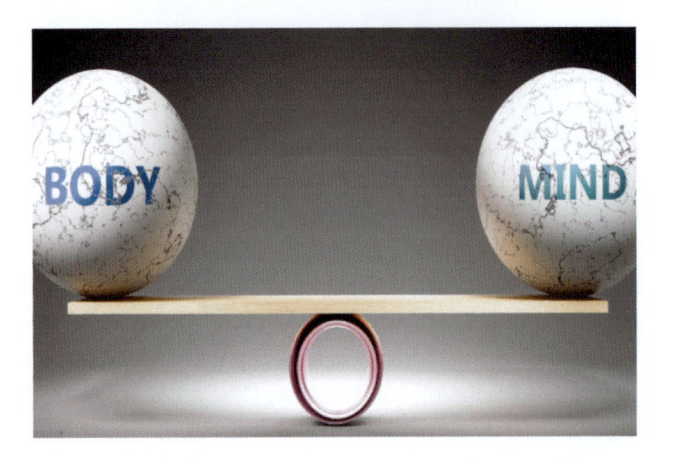

It's proven beyond all doubt that a healthy body helps with a healthy mind. And it's true. But do you know why? If not read on:

Everything is connected. What you do with and put into your body has a huge impact on your mental well being. Things like exercise, getting enough sleep, eating and drinking the right things for you, and not smoking, are just as important for your mind as they are for your body.

The converse is also true: mental health problems can affect your physical health. Low mood, depression, stress, anxiety, panic disorder etc can cause a multitude of physical issues such as high blood pressure, rheumatoid arthritis, headache/migraine, Crohn's Disease, irritable bowel syndrome, ulcers, eczema, psoriasis, loss of appetite, loss of weight, increased appetite, obesity, insomnia etc…the list goes on.

And the science behind it? When you exercise, chemical changes take place in your brain including neural growth, reduced inflammation and new electrical activity patterns, that enhance your mood and promote feelings of calm and well being. In addition, hormones known as endorphins that make you feel 'happier' and increase your energy levels are produced. These include serotonin, dopamine and noradrenaline.

This state, often referred to as a 'natural high', remains with you for a few hours after your exercise has finished. If you work out regularly, those natural highs blend into one another and you end up feeling good most of the time.

The same endorphins also stimulate the growth of new brain cells, which help prevent age-related decline – particularly important if you've reached your half century.

When exercise becomes a habit, the mental health benefits cumulatively increase to the point where exercise can be used and (even prescribed by a doctor as a 'medicine') for diagnosed conditions such as depression, anxiety, Attention Deficit Hyperactivity Disorder (ADHD) and Post Traumatic Stress Disorder (PTSD). It can also help boost your self esteem, confidence, keep you mentally sharp, mentally resilient and enhance your outlook on life in general.

In addition, the simple act of exerting yourself helps to relax the muscles after you've finished which, in turn, relieves tension in the body. Since the body and mind are so closely linked, when your body feels better, your mind does to.

And the good news is, you don't have to spend hours doing exercise to get the mental health benefits. As per the government advice, 30 minutes of moderate exercise five times a week is enough (even then you can choose to break it down into smaller segments e.g. 2 x 15 minutes).

Neither do you have to make exercise a solitary pastime. Much research has been done into the benefits of group exercise – either within a class or sport scenario, or just linking up with a family member or friend.

What matters is that you're socially connecting with a wider community. This on its own is good for your mental health. The fact you've got things in common with others could, over time, lead to a support network. Everyone knows, it's good to talk, particularly if you're feeling mentally or emotionally vulnerable.

42

LEARN HOW TO OVERCOME BARRIERS TO EXERCISE

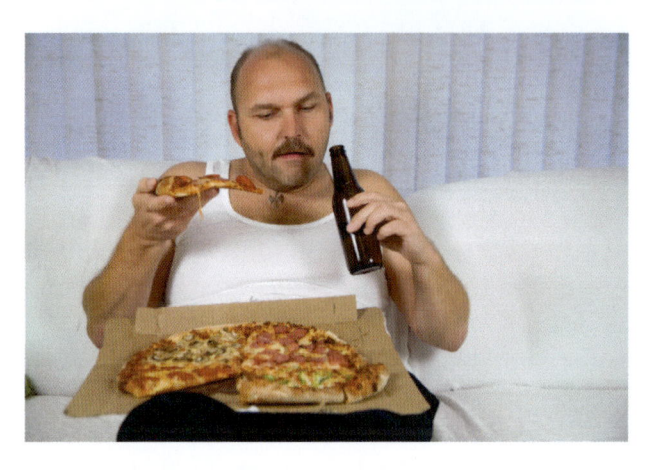

I know, I get it, you don't want to exercise. You're tired, you've had a long day at work, you've got a headache and you can think of scores of things you'd rather do - like your tax return, your ironing, or cleaning a blocked drain! In fact there's nothing you want to do less than get hot and sweaty while jiggling about.

So, what do you do? Well, most people go with the voice in their head telling them to opt out. They convince themselves they'll do it tomorrow/the weekend/some other time, and flop into a chair with a beer and a takeaway because it's an easier, more pleasurable option. (the body is also evolutionarily programmed to take the course of least resistance). These are the sort of people who haven't chosen to make exercise a priority and therefore haven't got a habit to stick to. The solution is simple - give yourself permission to make exercise a priority and then decide how best you're going to make it a habit. Experts say it takes between 18 and 254 days to form a habit. Everyone will be different because it depends on that person's motivation, personality and difficulty of the habit. Then, on average, it takes 66 days for a habit to become automatic behaviour.

Interestingly, the thing about habit, is that if you make it part of your everyday life and do it without question, something you previously thought of as out of the ordinary or unpleasant, slowly becomes something you want to do because it makes you feel 'normal.' That's the trick, make your habit a norm. Make exercise a norm.

That's not to say you won't come up against barriers and you may still find yourself making excuses not to exercise, but here are a few examples and how to deal with them:

I haven't got time:
Make time. Get up earlier, go to bed later, delete something else in your life that isn't a priority and substitute it with exercise.

I'm too tired/I've got no energy:
It might sound counterintuitive, but the more exercise you do, the more energy you're likely to have. Without exercise, you may have no energy at all whilst feeling fatigued and sluggish.

This is because exercise delivers oxygen and nutrients to tissue that improves the efficiency of your heart and lungs, which makes everyday activity feel easier. So, create an exercise-energy cycle and you'll be raring to go from morning to night.

I'm bored of exercise:
Try new things – a different type of workout, a different sport, a different location, use different equipment, sign up for fitness classes you've never done before and, crucially, set yourself new goals.

The weather's bad:
Exercise indoors or choose activities that aren't affected by the weather, e.g. indoor swimming, gym sessions or online fitness classes.

I'm travelling on business/going on a holiday etc:
Research accommodation before you book to ensure the facilities available are suitable for your exercise needs.

I can no longer afford my gym membership/personal trainer etc:
Many forms of exercise are free – running for example. Adapt your plan to suit your purse.

I've exercised in the past and failed to keep it up:
Re-evaluate what went wrong and change it. Look at your goals and

perhaps change them, but make the new ones realistic.

I'm too lazy:
Work *with* your nature, not against it. So, plan exercise at times of the day when you have most motivation or energy. Or, just decide you don't want to be that lazy person anymore.

I'm too self conscious about the way I look:
Avoid other people, exercise at home, or adopt a 'sod them' attitude. It's worth remembering that in places like gyms, everyone is so busy worrying about what they look like themselves, they haven't got time to focus on you. Honestly!

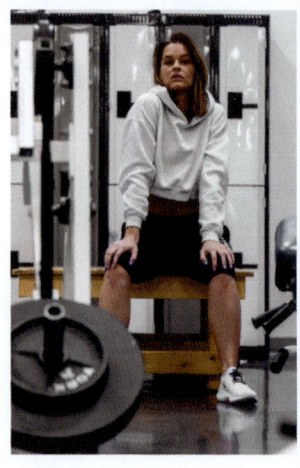

Adopt a 'sod them' attitude

43

FIND INSPIRATION, BUT BE CAREFUL HOW YOU USE SOCIAL MEDIA

There's no harm in having role models or people you look up to. It's normal and can be useful. But do not rule out the everyday people you come across such as the woman across the road who lost two stone last year, goes running every Sunday and now looks ten years younger. You're both around 55, your children go to university and you sometimes bump into her in the supermarket. If you decide to take a leaf out of her book and embark on a health and fitness regime, that's helpful because you're comparing like with like and she inspired you in a positive, achievable way.

If, however, you scroll through social media for hours looking at pictures of perfectly formed, young women doing athletic things on an exotic beach in a tiny bikini, then that's unhelpful because, let's face it, you're never going to look like her and you've been influenced in a negative way that made you feel inadequate.

HEALTH WARNING:

Image-oriented social media is bad for your health. Why torture yourself looking at pictures of other people when many of those pictures do not reflect reality? The woman in them is probably a fitness model, the picture was probably the 'money shot' out of hundreds taken, and it's almost certainly been edited to within an inch of its life.

With middle age comes perspective and wisdom. By now you should be able to accept that it's not possible to be someone else and there's no point trying.

Instead, focus on being the best possible version of yourself and work within your limitations so that results are in line with who you are. Sure, use social media for ideas and a good laugh, but don't look at pictures that are going to make you feel bad about your body or your life. And, if you're following someone whose images do that, just unfollow them.

I don't see any harm in respecting people in the public eye who have clearly worked their butts off to defy age. Some notable ones over the age of 50 include: Jane Fonda, 83, Madonna, 60, Carol Vorderman, 60, Jennifer Aniston, 51, Davina McCall, 53, Tom Cruise, 58, George Clooney, 59, Brad Pitt, 57 and yoga fanatic Sting, 69.

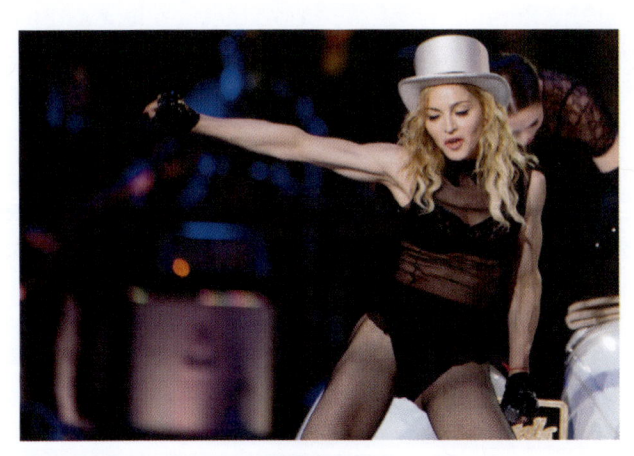

Madonna

44

WORK HARD - BUT BE KIND TO YOURSELF

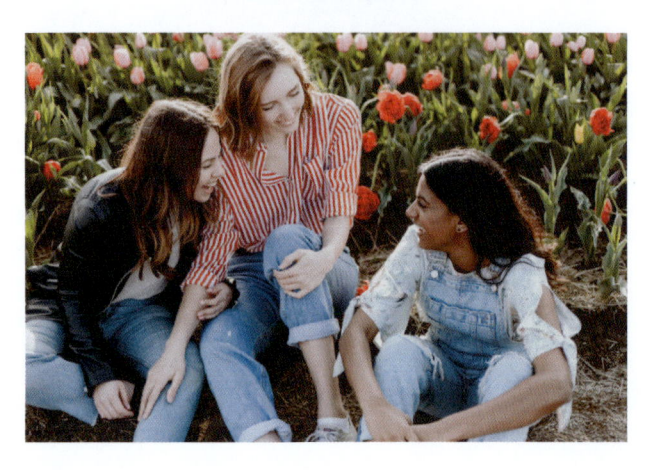

I mentioned at the beginning of the book that it's just as possible for you to reach your health and fitness potential as it is for a 20-year-old. Everything is relative, of course, but the common factor whatever your age is this: to get great results you must work hard. If you work in a half-hearted way, you'll get mediocre results.

I honestly believe if you're going to put effort into something, you might as well give 100%. This applies to changing the way you eat to exercise (and life in general).

'No pain, no gain,' is a cliché but I'm afraid it's true much of the time. It's not easy swapping that bar of chocolate for an apple, it's hard to complete that third set of bicep curls when your muscles are screaming at you to stop.

But if you do — and keep doing these sorts of things — you will see results both mentally and physically. Not only will your body and health change for the better, but you'll build a level of self-respect, pride and resilience that you never thought possible. You're not born with these characteristics; they have to be earned. If you work hard enough to acquire them, you'll find they are rewards in themselves, but that shouldn't stop you finding other things to keep you going. So, relax, treat yourself.

Although you should choose a treat that appeals to you, I warn against making it food.

You don't have to earn food. Food is your body's right. Food is essential for survival and food is fuel for the day's activities — including exercise. Try and view it this way, rather than a way of spoiling yourself or an emotional crutch. That's not to say you shouldn't occasionally have that bar of chocolate at the end of the week because you really, really want it. And it certainly doesn't mean never going out to dinner and such like.

In fact, I recommend you pro-actively incorporate these sorts of treats into your regime from time to time, because they help motivated, they're acts of self-kindness and they're not going to de-rail your progress if they're the exception rather than the rule.

DO NOT do deals with yourself like: 'if I cut my calories by 100 a day, on Sunday I can scoff two Mars Bars and a glass of wine.' That's unhealthy behaviour and, over time, could lead to disordered eating.

Rewards don't have to be things, they can be experiences, e.g. a trip to the cinema, a long soak in the bath, reading a book in a coffee shop, getting your hair done, practising yoga, etc.

In modern parlance, being kind to yourself is known as **self-care.** The precise definition is: the practice of consciously doing things that preserve or improve your mental or physical health.

The younger generation take self-care very seriously because they've grown up in an environment where it's normal and encouraged. They know that mental and physical health are linked and that both need to be nurtured. They don't schedule rewards into their life, they do things on an on-going basis that promote well-being.

They don't restrict it to themselves either. They practice self-care with their friends. They share and emote with them and allow themselves to be vulnerable with other people. They do not consider any of this self-indulgent or selfish, they see it as vital - and with good reason. All the research and studies into mental health, show that this way of living beats good old fashioned stiff upper lip and being hard on yourself.

So work hard, but also take a leaf out of Generation Z's book and care for yourself and others to promote health and happiness.

45
ACCEPT THERE WILL BE SETBACKS, BUT KEEP CALM AND CARRY ON!

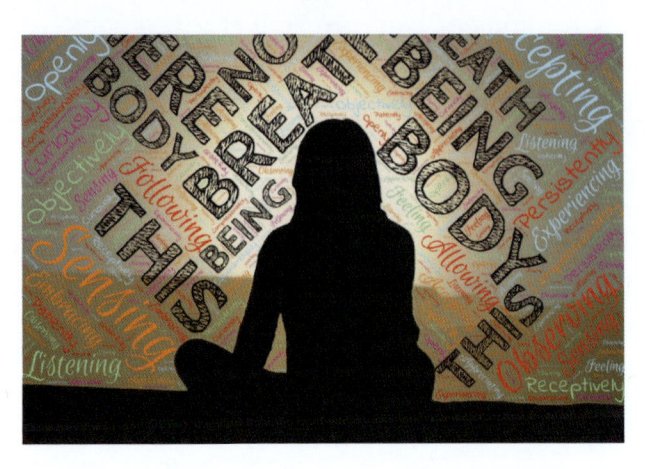

Setbacks, mistakes, disappointments, complications, knock-backs. They're part of everyday life. Progression isn't linear and you simply have to learn from things that go wrong.

Where weight loss and exercise are concerned, there are two types of setback — the longer term **'plateau'** type and the short term **'whoops'** type. I give you examples:

- **Plateau for weight loss** — you stop losing weight because you've become complacent about food choices. You're anxious on an on-going basis.
- **Plateau for exercise** — you're not exercising as regularly as you once did and you're getting out of breath sooner when you do. You're anxious on an on-going basis.
- **Whoops! for weight loss** – you binge on takeaway fried food and feel guilty for a short period of time.
- **Whoops! for exercise** – you skip the gym because you can't be bothered to go and feel guilty for a short period of time.

Whether the setback is on-going or a one-off behaviour, the **first** thing to do is NOT beat yourself up over it or punish yourself with sanctions (so no starving yourself or spending three hours in the gym the next day). You're human, you're allowed to mess up and maybe there was a good reason why it happened — perhaps because you were ravenously hungry.

Setbacks are normal and should be expected. You must not let them define you. Rather, learn from them to prevent similar occurrences. Ask yourself if maybe your goals are unrealistic and that's what your body is trying to tell you through sabotage.

Secondly, get back on the horse. Setbacks can indicate a loss of control, so it's important to regain that control before you convince yourself it's too late. This can mean anything from simply reverting to the old habits and behaviours that were working for you, to re-planning your strategy and setting new goals.

Thirdly, try not to have an 'all or nothing' mentality. One or two mistakes will not ruin everything, in fact they may not have any negative effect. Keep lapses in perspective and try to look at the bigger picture. Remind yourself that health and fitness is a lifestyle not a goal to be reached and then discarded. Moreover, if you want to make the lifestyle sustainable, you have to allow yourself NOT to be perfect. Also, acknowledge that there will be highs and lows but that living somewhere in the middle is OK.

And **lastly**, don't be afraid to ask for support — be it from a friend, family member or professional. Asking for help is not a sign of weakness, it's a sign of strength. It demonstrates your determination to improve yourself.

46

PRACTICE MINDFUL - NOT MINDLESS - EXERCISE AND EATING

Mindfulness is the basic human ability to be fully present, aware of where we are and what we're doing, while not being reactive or overwhelmed by outside influences. It's a state of mind rather than a trait of character, and although it doesn't need to be conjured up, there are techniques to access it. There are multiple proven benefits of practising mindfulness in everyday life. They include: feeling more content and calm, stress and anxiety reduction, improved sleep, enhanced focus and increased productivity.

The last benefit is the main one where mindful exercise is concerned. Think about it, whether you're running, swimming, playing bowls or skiing, the more you're able to focus on the activity, the better at it you're likely to be. This is for a number of reasons, e.g. because you're concentrating on your technique, because you're looking at a timer in order to push yourself harder, or because you're simply 'in the zone' and serious about the task in hand.

Also, not being distracted by things like blaring music in a gym, means you have the mental space to focus on the things that are important to you in life — including the exercise you're actually doing. With regards eating, if you're doing something else whilst eating, the chances are you won't even remember it, let alone appreciate the food. So, switch off the TV, sit at a table, serve up your food on a nice plate and think about what you're doing — chew the food well, savour the taste, experience the sensation of it being digested and be grateful for the pleasure it's hopefully bringing you. This is, of course, particularly pertinent if you're on any sort of 'diet' and controlling your food intake.

The process of mindful eating starts long before you take the first mouthful. If you're focussed and present where your diet is concerned, you're more likely to make the sort of food choices that benefit the regime you've chosen. Mindless eating can often mean fast eating — which isn't good for you. When you slow everything down, it aids digestion because enzymes are stimulated that break down the food efficiently. Mindfulness is not the same thing as meditation, but it has similar qualities, one of them being your mind unwinds and de-clutters; the other is that you're required to concentrate on your breathing.

To start the mindfulness process, do just that — concentrate on the sensation of your breaths, how the air feels in your nose, mouth and chest as you inhale and the difference when you exhale. Take deep breaths from below your diaphragm and notice your belly and chest rising and falling. It's inevitable that your mind will start wandering. It's not a problem, just rein it back in and re-focus on your breathing. The difference between it and hypnosis/meditation where exercise and eating are concerned, is that it's OK to have two behaviours running consecutively.

Mindfulness is simple, but that doesn't make it easy. Like any other skill it must be practiced and the more you do it, the more you'll be storing up the benefits which you'll experience over time.

47

EAT GOOD-MOOD FOODS AND FOODS THAT NOURISH THE BRAIN

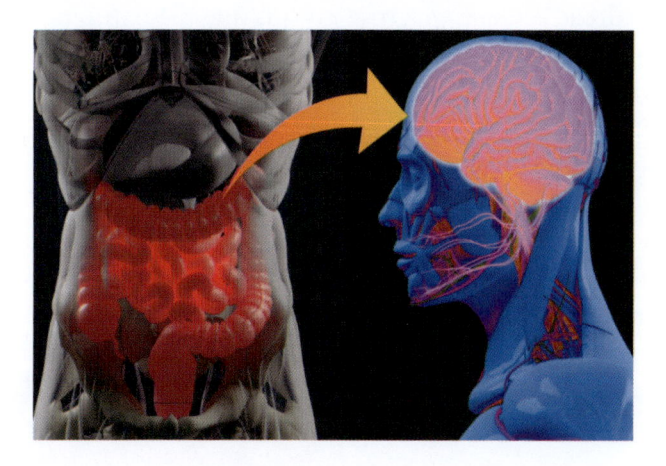

Mental health is very much in the public arena nowadays. It's discussed, dissected and delved into in a bid to help everybody improve their own well-being. That's a huge and much needed development. But mental health isn't just about feeling stable, balanced and able to cope with life's challenges, it also refers to the physical health of the brain as an organ — something few people think about.

Brain health is a relatively new strand of science that investigates what we can do to prevent the brain deteriorating as we get older. Researchers have already found evidence that certain aspects of brain ageing — such as short-term memory loss — start many years before symptoms show.

For many over 50s, those symptoms will already have started, e.g. you asked somebody their name and 30 seconds later you can't remember it.

Science suggests that you can slow down these processes — even after they've started — by including certain foods in your diet. There is also proof that some foods can boost your mood and your mental health in general.

This is because the brain and the gut are connected both physically and bio-chemically in several ways, including via the nervous and immune systems. This connection is known as the **brain-gut-axis.**

This is why you can get 'butterflies in your tummy' when you're nervous about something or you can feel sick in times of trouble/challenge. The connection between the two is influenced by the millions of microbes in the gut known as the **microbiome.** The healthier it is, the healthier you and your brain are. The most efficient way to keep your gut healthy is by trying to maintain a healthy balance among the hundreds of different species of bacteria in your gut. There are two ways to do this — helping the microbes already there to grow by giving them foods they like — *prebiotic* — and adding living microbes to the mix — *probiotic*.

Prebiotic rich foods include:
Carrots, turnip, cabbage, sweet potato, asparagus, artichokes, onions, leeks, raw garlic and chia seeds.

Probiotic rich foods include:
Yoghurt and brined vegetables such as sauerkraut, kefir (a fermented milk drink) kimchi, pickles and spirulina.

Other foods which can help mental health are:

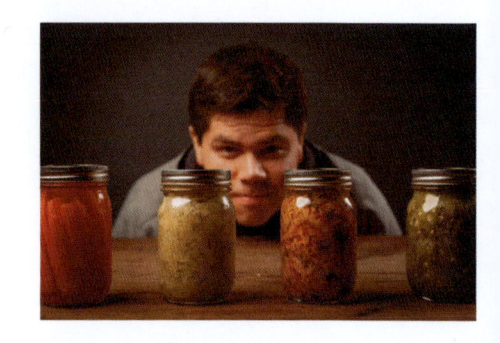

Serotonin-rich foods (for mood, sleep, pain and craving control):
Eggs, turkey, seafood, chickpeas, nuts and seeds, quinoa and dark chocolate.

Dopamine-rich foods (for motivation):
Lentils, fish, lamb, beef, eggs, pumpkin and sesame seeds and high protein veggies like broccoli and spinach.

Antioxidant-rich foods (to help protect cells — including those in the brain):
All berries, pomegranate, kidney beans, parsley, cocoa powder, walnuts, olive oil and green tea.

Spices (for focus and attention):
Turmeric, saffron, peppermint, cinnamon

Magnesium-rich foods (for anxiety):
Pumpkin and sunflower seeds, almonds, cashews, Swiss Chard, sesame seeds and spinach.

Vitamin B6, B12, folate-rich foods (for cell growth and nervous system maintenance):
Salmon, sardines, tuna, liver, soy and almond milk, beef, eggs, cabbage, bok-choy, cauliflower, bell peppers and parsley.

Zinc rich foods (cell and immune system protection):
Oysters, shiitake mushrooms, beef, lamb, liver, avocado, hemp seeds, ricotta cheese and yoghurt.

We know that diet and exercise are two of the most important tools you can use to improve your mental and physical health, it should not be overlooked, however, that excessive behaviours in these areas are likely to be bad for your mental health. A sign that you've taken things too far is if you're prioritising diet and exercise over all other things and you're changing your life to accommodate the situation, e.g. not eating out socially.

If enthusiasm has morphed into obsession and the compulsion to stick to a particular type of diet and exercise regime is so overwhelming you can't stop, it could mean you're in the grip of an eating disorder.

Eating disorders are serious mental health conditions that can have life-long and life-limiting consequences. In fact, anorexia nervosa has the highest mortality rate of ANY mental illness. Eating disorders are also widely misunderstood. They aren't just 'diets gone wrong', and they're not just about food, eating or over-exercise, they are a complex type of addiction which often serve as a coping mechanism or a way to feel in control of circumstances or feelings.

They also take many different forms — some of which have a name or label, some of which don't. The main ones are:

Anorexia:
Sufferers try to eat as little as possible in order to drop to the lowest weight possible. The disease is characterised by using techniques to get rid of food that has been consumed. This can include purging through self-induced vomiting, excessive exercise and laxative abuse.

Bulimia:
Sufferers are caught in a binge-purge cycle. This means they'll consume a large amount of food and to compensate may stop eating for a while and/or get rid of it in the same way as anorexics.

Binge Eating Disorder:
Similar to bulimia but not normally with the purging aspect.

OSFED (other specified feeding or eating disorder):
An umbrella term to describe disordered eating that doesn't fit into the other three categories — even though *some* of the symptoms may be the same (e.g. someone may drastically restrict food but remain a normal weight)

If you think that because you're over 50 you're immune to developing an eating disorder, think again. It's an erroneous stereotype that only young women get eating disorders. They can affect any one of any age, gender, race or social class. The issues that cause them in young people do not simply disappear as one gets older. In fact one of the main triggers in the young — a shift in self-identity during adolescence — is particularly common in middle age as life changes due to events like children leaving home or because retirement looms.

48

IF YOUR ENTHUSIASM FOR DIET AND EXERCISE HAS BEOME A COMPULSION, SEEK MEDICAL HELP

While it's true to say that funding for the treatment of eating disorders in the UK is woefully lacking, it does exist. The only way to access it on the NHS is via your GP, so book an appointment as soon as you can.

Treatments will vary depending on what type of eating disorder you have and how extreme it is, but it will almost certainly involve some sort of 'talking therapy'.

49

KEEP MENTALLY ACTIVE TO PREVENT COGNITIVE DECLINE AND TO BOOST MENTAL HEALTH

Your brain is a muscle, just like any other muscle in the body. It therefore follows that to keep it fit and healthy, you can — and should — exercise it, like any other muscle.

Studies show that mental decline is NOT an inevitable part of ageing and people who lead intellectually stimulating lives *can* be protected from conditions like dementia. All this is increasingly important as we age because brain cells die at an alarmingly quick rate and you can't get them back.

Staying mentally active doesn't mean going all-studious just because you're over 50. It means finding enjoyable things to do that stimulate your mind. Here are a few ideas:

- Read more — a newspaper, a book, a blog…anything
- Do a daily crossword, puzzle or quiz
- Play a brain stimulating game such as chess or Scrabble
- Do mental arithmetic rather than using a calculator
- Do a jigsaw puzzle
- Colour in. Adult colouring books are all the rage
- Start an adult education course. Most colleges do them.
- Take up a new interest or hobby — e.g. learning to play a musical instrument or joining a tai chi class
- Stay socially active — preferably in person, rather than online — and have good conversation/debate
- Go out more (with or without a friend). Many stimulating places are free e.g. art galleries
- Change everyday things and routines, maybe take a different route to work, get a new haircut, try an alternative supermarket, etc.
- Go outside when you wouldn't normally. Walk in the snow or the pelting rain. Why not?

Do some or all of these things — along with your everyday activities — and not only will you be busier, but you'll also be more engaged with yourself, others and life in general. This may well boost your mood, give you a more positive outlook and provide you with purpose in life — the types of things that generally help improve mental health.

We now come to the last point of the book and it's an all-encompassing one that highlights ways of living that should lead to a better quality and quantity of life.

PART FOUR

LIFESTYLE

50
TAKE THE FOLLOWING LIFESTYLE ADVICE

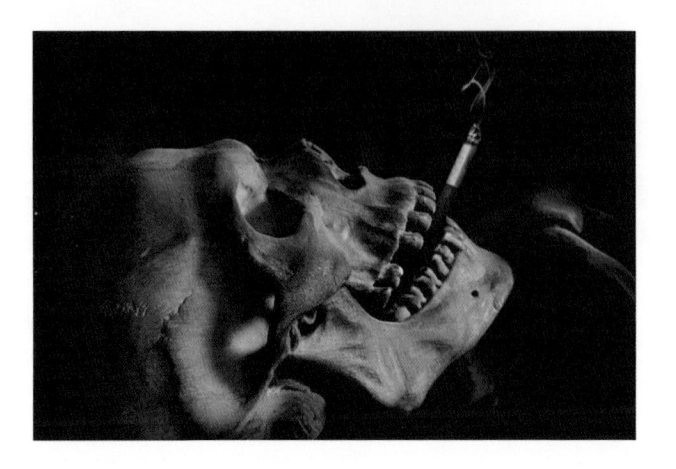

If you ignore all the other guidance in this book, do not ignore this: **DON'T SMOKE – EVER.** And, if you do, give up now.

The World Health Organisation describes it as:

> *"An epidemic, one of the biggest public health threats the world has ever faced."*

Fact:
Smoking will kill approximately half the people who do it as well as people who don't (through second hand smoke). There are a million reasons why you shouldn't smoke, and this book isn't long enough to list them all. Needless to say, it's the most dangerous legal thing you can inflict on yourself.

Sleep:
Everyone knows sleep is important, but few appreciate *how* important.

Most people think the significance relates to how much you get, when what matters more is the quality rather than the quantity. This applies whatever your age, but even more so after middle age, when you're in a physiological decline.

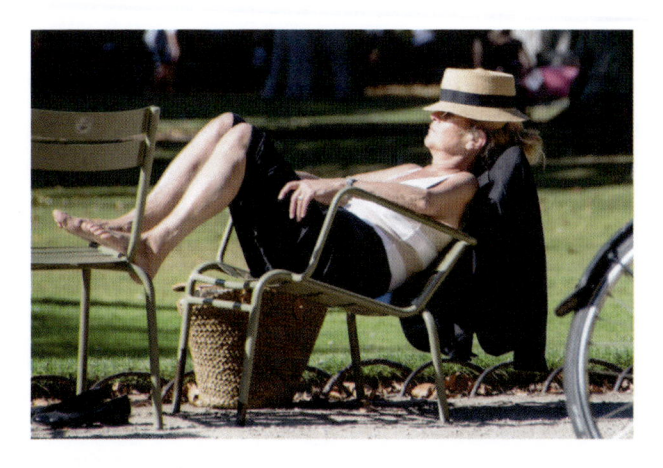

We spend about a third of our life asleep. Just like a lack of food and water, without it we would die. The theory has been tested scientifically on rats who can last without sleep for around two weeks. The longest recorded time for a human is just under 11 days.

Sleep and health work symbiotically — poor sleep can lead to poor health and poor health can lead to poor sleep. The odd bad night's sleep can make you feel tired and irritable the next day, but it won't harm your long-term health. Regular poor quality sleep can have a huge impact on your health putting you at risk of developing serious medical conditions like heart disease, diabetes, high blood pressure and obesity. In addition, it can detrimentally affect your mental health in terms of your thoughts, emotions and behaviour.

Most people need around eight hours of good quality sleep per night to function fully. Good quality means falling asleep within approximately 20 minutes, not waking up more than once for a short time and not having persistent disruptive dreams. Most people do not get eight hours and they do not function properly — although they're unlikely to realise this.

Here are 8 reasons why enough good quality sleep is essential for good health:

1) Good sleep keeps your heart healthy. Interrupted sleep stimulates part of the nervous system responsible for producing 'fight or flight' hormones which, in turn, lead to an increase in blood pressure. The extra strain on the body in general — and the heart specifically — can lead to coronary heart disease and stroke.

2) Poor sleep is linked to being overweight. This is because poor sleep interrupts the natural balance of hormones that are linked to appetite and metabolism. This includes higher levels of ghrelin, the hormone that stimulates appetite, and lower levels of leptin, an appetite suppressant.

3) Sleep improves your immune function. Which protects against everyday conditions such as the common cold. It also enables you to fight disease. This is because while you sleep, your body builds and repairs itself by making new tissue.

4) Sleep deprivation affects blood sugar and reduces insulin sensitivity. In less than a week of deprived sleep you can become pre-diabetic, Over time, fully diabetic.

5) Lack of good quality sleep can be a contributory factor in mental health issues. Including, depression and anxiety. A study showed that 90% of people with depression also suffered from poor quality sleep or insomnia.

6) Sleep improves your brain function. This includes cognition, concentration, productivity, performance, memory and problem-solving skills.

7) Sleep enables you to function normally in terms of meeting everyday demands including, exercise and strenuous activity. This is because the body repairs and rejuvenates itself when in a deep state of rest.

8) Good sleep reduces stress. When you're stressed, the body produces a hormone called cortisol which stays in your bloodstream and keeps you stressed. Good sleep relaxes the systems of the body responsible for producing it.

There are many things you can do to help you get to sleep AND stay asleep. Here are some of them:

- Avoid caffeine, nicotine, and alcohol too near bedtime. They are stimulants that may keep you awake
- Avoid screen time before you go to bed — put away your phone, laptop etc at least an hour before you retire

- Keeping physically active in the day will tire you out to the extent where your body needs sleep to recover
- Try something relaxing before bedtime e.g. yoga, or having a warm bath
- Use relaxation techniques such as meditation, deep breathing or ASMR (autonomous sensory meridian response) — the fashionable practice of getting physical, relaxing, tingling sensations through audio-visual triggers such as someone whispering, tapping, or brushing.
- Cool down the temperature — open a window, wear lightweight nightclothes, etc.
- Use essential oils — such as lavender — on your body or pillow.

Don't bother counting sheep, it doesn't work — studies show it's too boring to distract you enough from the types of things that keep you awake at night — namely the stresses and strains of the day.

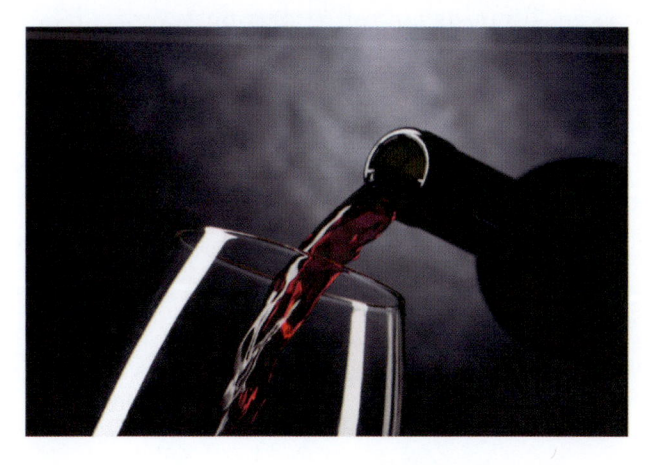

Alcohol:
Let's be clear, a bit of alcohol is not going to kill you. In fact, research shows that some alcohol in moderation is good for your health, e.g., red wine.

However…a lot of alcohol on a regular basis might just kill you. Be sensible. If you want a drink have one, but keep your intake moderate and keep it under control. So, no binge drinking because it happens to be the weekend and don't drink every night.

A glass of red with your meal is fine, a bottle of red with your meal is not. The government says we shouldn't drink more than 14 units a week. This equates to 6 pints of average strength beer or 10 small glasses of low strength wine. This, of course, should be adhered to. But who measures out units at home and who's honest about their units when they go to their GP? The truth is, if you like a drink and you're not measuring out or counting units, then you're probably exceeding the advisory limit and you should probably cut down.

Checks and Screenings:
It's natural to become increasingly concerned about your health as you get older — even if you are seemingly fit and healthy and not overweight.

The good news is that there is a health 'MOT' which you can access free of charge via the NHS which will either put your mind at rest or flag up problems that can then be dealt with sooner rather than later. Called the **NHS Health Checklist**, it is available to anyone aged between 40 and 74 who does not have a pre-existing serious condition that is already being treated.

Once you're over 40, your GP surgery should invite you for one every five years — but if they don't, all you have to do is call your surgery and request one.

Whether you get other checks via the NHS or access them privately, the following types are available and recommended once you're over 50.

Blood Pressure Check:

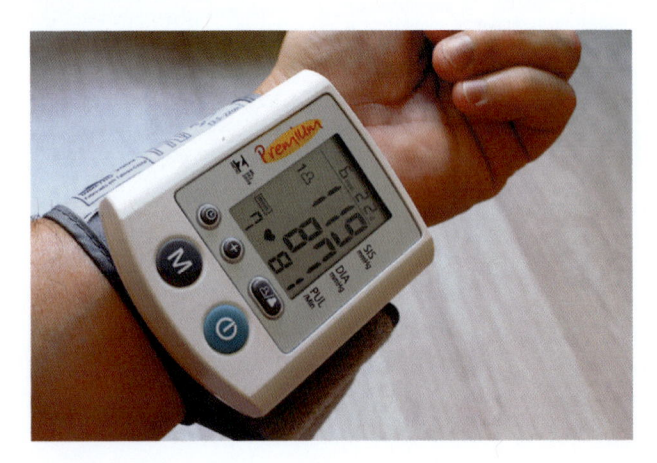

One of the problems of high blood pressure is that you only know you've got it if you have your blood pressure taken. There aren't obvious signs and symptoms. Normal blood pressure is from 100/70 to 120/80. The top number is your systolic measurement — the pressure at which your heart is pumping out blood through veins and arteries. The bottom number —

diastolic — is the pressure at which your heart is resting between beats. You can easily check it yourself by buying a cheap digital device.

Cholesterol Checks:
Cholesterol is a type of fat found in you blood. Your body needs it to function, but high levels can block your arteries which increases your risk of heart attacks and strokes.

Bowel Cancer Screening:
To be entitled to get this on the NHS you have to be over the age of 60. The test — involving a sample of your faeces – doesn't diagnose cancer, but it does detect signs of blood in your sample which would then lead to further diagnostic tests. Bowel cancer is the fourth most common cancer in the UK.

Breast Screening:
One in eight women in the UK will get breast cancer in her lifetime and it is the most common cancer in the UK. It mainly affects women over the age of 50 but men and young women can, and do, get it too. Women over the age of 50 should be invited to have a mammogram every five years by their local NHS. A mammogram is a type of x-ray which detects abnormalities of cells in the breast tissue. You should also check your own breasts (and chest and armpits) for changes in appearance, sensation and lumps.

Cervical Cancer Screening:
This is offered to women up to the age of 64 by the NHS. From the age of 25-49, every three years and from the age of 50-64, every five years. Around 3,000 cases of cervical cancer are diagnosed in the UK every year.

Abdominal Aortic Aneurysm Check:
An aortic aneurysm is a swelling in your aorta (the main blood vessel in your body). If it bursts, it can lead to a life threatening bleed in your stomach. Often there are no symptoms.
The condition is more prevalent in men than women and the NHS offers the test to males in their 65th year.

Skin Checks:
Whether you check yourself or visit a specialist clinic or your GP, keeping an eye on moles and certain types of skin lesions can help you to spot the first signs of skin cancer.

If an existing mole changes in appearance/colour or shape, you should seek medical attention.

Vaccinations:
People usually recover from illnesses such as flu, pneumonia or shingles without any ongoing consequences. In later life, however, they can cause major problems and can prove fatal. If you're over the age of 65, you can get a free flu jab every year on the NHS. If you're aged between 70-79 you can get a one-off shingles jab.

COVID-19 Vaccination:

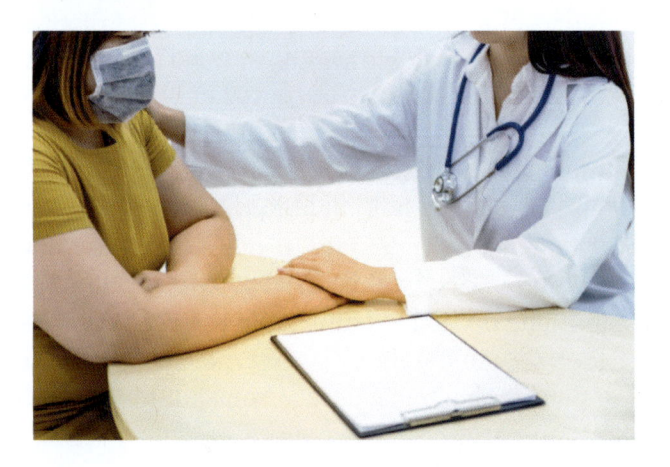

At the beginning of 2021 the Government produced a nine point priority list of those eligible for the vaccine in the first phase of the rollout. People over the age of 50 came in at number 9.

It's also worth mentioning, as this is a book about health, fitness and weight, that early on in the pandemic it emerged from NHS statistics that obesity is one of the major risk factors in contracting COVID-19. More disturbingly, being overweight increases your chance of dying from it by 40%.

AFTERWORD

That's it. I'm all advised-out. Over to you now. You've two choices: take my advice, follow the 50 steps and give yourself the chance of a better, longer life…or ignore my advice and use the book as a mat for a huge plate of junk food. If you're torn between the two, let me help you decide by posing a question:

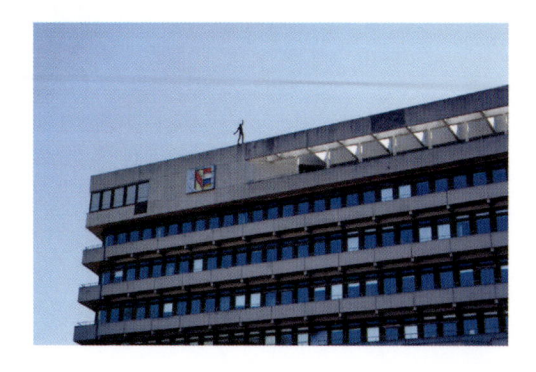

If I dared you to stand on the ledge of a high building would you do it?

The answer would almost certainly be no — because you know you'd probably fall and either seriously injure yourself or die. But, if you're over 50, fat and unfit and know this could seriously damage your health or kill you, why on earth wouldn't you apply the same logic and change the way you live?

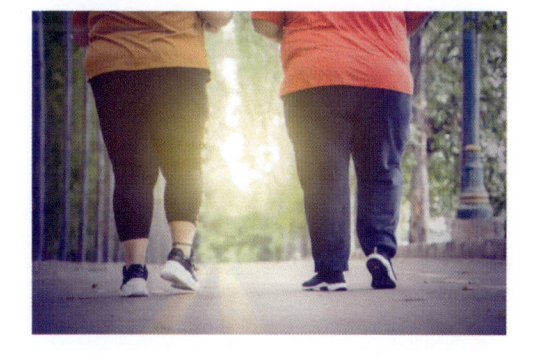

It's a no brainer…

"Over 50, fat and unfit?

You really are a bit of a twit;

you've read this book so now you see,

how much better your life could be."

Aylia Fox

www.foxthefitness.com

facebook.com/foxthefitness

twitter.com/aylia43

instagram.com/_fox.fitness_

Printed in Great Britain
by Amazon